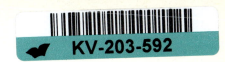

The Treatment of
Chronic Pain

The Treatment of
Chronic Pain

Edited by
Dr F. Dudley Hart

MTP
Medical and Technical Publishing Co Ltd

Published by

MTP
MEDICAL AND TECHNICAL
PUBLISHING CO LTD
PO Box 55, St Leonard's House,
St Leonardgate,
Lancaster, Lancs

ISBN 0 85200082 0

First Published 1974

Filmset by Technical Filmsetters Europe Ltd
and

Printed by The Garden City Press Limited,
Letchworth, Hertfordshire SG6 1JS

Contents

List of Contributors

F. Dudley Hart, M.D., F.R.C.P.
Consultant Physician, Westminster Hospital, London, SW1

E. C. Huskisson, B.Sc., M.B., M.R.C.P.
Senior Medical Registrar, St Bartholomew's Hospital
London, EC1

Stanley A. Feldman, M.B., B.S.
Consultant Anesthetist, Westminster Hospital, London, SW1

Thomas S. Szasz, M.D.
Professor of Psychiatry, State University of New York
Upstate Medical Center, Syracuse, N.Y.

Gerald Westbury, M.B., M.R.C.P., F.R.C.S.
Consultant Surgeon, Westminster Hospital, London, SW1

James C. White, M.D.
Emeritus Professor of Surgery, Harvard Medical School
former chief of Neurosurgical Service,
Massachusetts General Hospital, Boston, Mass.

Foreword

Despite the fact that pain is the central theme running through all branches of medicine and surgery and is the main reason for our patients coming to see us, relatively little has been written of its long-term control. Of all pain it is the chronic unremitting variety that is the most difficult to ease effectively and to control adequately. To relieve what has been called 'the long pain' has been the aim of the six authors in this book. In such a huge subject we have not tried to cover all aspects of therapy, but have merely aimed to discuss how we, the authors, set out to control chronic pain in some of its more common forms by drugs and by surgery and other methods. We have not attempted to discuss pain control by other means, such as manipulation or acupuncture. The authors are Physicians (two), Surgeons (two), anesthetist (one) and Psychiatrist (one). Each chapter is individual and complete in itself and therefore there is some, though relatively little, overlap. We hope that medical students as well as General Practitioners and Medical and Surgical specialists may find something of interest in these pages, though they are written essentially for the General Practitioner and final year medical students. And, finally, the Editor is immensely grateful to his Collaborators for their magnificent co-operation and to the Publishers for their ready help at all times.

F. DUDLEY HART
Westminster Hospital,
London, SW1

1

Pain: Mechanisms
and Measurement

E. C. Huskisson

Pain is an everyday experience, a feature of psychological as well as physical illness, an advantage in health and a disadvantage in disease; few can ignore it. For doctors it is the complaint of their patients; two of every three patients seeking medical help have pain (Suchman, 1965; Devine and Merskey, 1965). For patients it is the complaint from which relief is desired; most are unconcerned with laboratory tests and measure the success of treatment only in terms of the symptom, pain. For these reasons, pain has attracted the interest of doctors, who wanted to know the mechanism of its production in the hope of interfering with the process. The ability to measure pain is essential for scientific study of the phenomenon as well as for accurate evaluation of treatment designed to relieve it.

Pain is a sensation which we all recognize even if we cannot define it. As such it has aroused interest from earliest times. Keele (1962) has reviewed historical concepts attempting to explain the localization and mechanism of pain sensation. For Aristotle, the heart situated in the center of the body was the seat of sensation, receiving ripples from the periphery and transmitting them in the blood vessels. Plato suggested that pain was the result of the violent actions of the four elements, earth, air, fire and water, on the soul. Though the central nervous system was discovered in about 300 BC, it was not until the nineteenth century AD that further progress was made as a result of careful observation and experiment. Since that time, knowledge of pain mechanisms has developed in two separate ways, one concerned with the physiological mechanisms, the anatomical, physical and chemical requirements for the production of the sensation of pain, the other concerned with psychological mechanisms. The beginning of progress was the discovery by Bell that the posterior nerve root was a specific organ of sensation; this led Muller to postulate that individual nervous pathways carried particular sensations, the beginning of the search for the 'pain pathway'. Later the surgeon was able to study the effects of dividing pathways and the physiologist to demonstrate the electrical activity of individual nerve fibers.

The mechanism of pain; anatomical, physiological and biochemical considerations

THE RECEPTOR
Von Frey (1895) described specific nerve endings for each of four cutaneous modalities, including pain for which the receptor was a free nerve ending. He showed that pain spots could be identified, and at these spots, other modalities such as touch were not perceived. Woollard *et al.* (1940) studied nerve endings in the rabbit ear and showed that responses interpreted as indicating that the animals felt pain were produced by stimulation of free endings of non-medullated and finer medullated nerve fibers in the deeper layers of the epidermis. Though the free nerve endings are capable of responding to noxious stimuli, though not necessarily exclusively so, combined clinical and histological studies have failed to support the assignation of the other modalities such as temperature to a specific end-organ. Iggo (1972) argues that specific pain receptors must exist since some isolated nerve fibers respond only to certain types of noxious stimuli.

CHEMOSENSITIVITY
Keele and Armstrong (1964) showed that there were chemosensitive pain receptors. They applied a cantharidin plaster to human skin producing a blister, the top of which could be removed leaving an exposed area thought to contain pain receptors. It was then possible to demonstrate that some naturally occurring substances such as bradykinin, which is involved in the process of acute inflammation, were capable of inducing pain at very low concentrations. Pain could also be produced by hydrogen or potassium ions, histamine,

5-hydroxytryptamine, acetylcholine and various peptides, but not adrenalin or nor-adrenalin. Recent evidence suggests that prostaglandin E_1 is able to sensitize the pain receptor to the action of chemical mediators and other stimuli such as pressure, though it is not itself a pain-producing substance except in very high concentrations. Ferreira (1972) infused prostaglandin E_1 subdermally in human volunteers and showed that this increased sensitivity to bradykinin or histamine; pain was also elicited by slight pressure over the infusion site. This effect of prostaglandin E_1 also suggests a mechanism of action for peripherally-acting analgesics such as aspirin; Vane (1971) showed that aspirin inhibits prostaglandin synthetase, preventing the formation of prostaglandins. Relief of pain may be produced by the absence of the sensitizing effect of prostaglandin E_1 on pain receptors.

NERVE FIBERS
Bishop (1946) produced evidence that each sensory modality was associated with activity in sensory fibers within size ranges whose maxima at least were characteristic; for pain, peak activity was found in large rapidly-conducting myelinated A delta fibers and the small slow-conducting unmyelinated C fibers. These fibers are not specific for the sensation of pain; Douglas and Ritchie (1957) showed that C fibers could respond to non-noxious mechanical stimuli such as light touch. Hensel *et al.* (1960) studied isolated single C fiber preparations and showed that though some fibers may be specific for one mode of stimulation, others can respond to different types of stin.uli.

TRACTS AND COLUMNS
The pathways of pain fibers inside the spinal cord and central nervous system have been mapped largely as a result of surgical experience in the relief of pain, aided by the effects of accidental injuries. McCarty and Drake (1956) summarize surgical experience; structures apparently involved in pain transmission or perception include the dorsal root, the lateral spino-thalamic tract, the thalamus and the prefrontal cortex. Surgical lesions of these structures modify pain but do not necessarily abolish it; in fact such lesions may cause pain. Other structures are involved indirectly, for example the sympathetic nervous system.

GATE THEORY

Melzack and Wall (1965) proposed a unifying theory of pain mechanism, the gate theory. The gate is situated anatomically in cells of the substantia gelatinosa, which are found in dorsal horns throughout the spinal cord. The first central transmission or T cells send sensory information to higher centers after it has passed through the gate. Sensory information is also transmitted centrally in the dorsal columns and, after processing, can influence the gate by way of descending tracts; this constitutes the central control mechanism.

The gate theory sets out to explain a number of observations concerning pain mechanisms. Pain is mediated by a group of large fibers and a group of small fibers. Volleys of nerve impulses in large fibers are initially effective in activating groups of T cells in the spinal cord of the cat; later this effect is reduced by an inhibitory mechanism. Volleys in small fibers activate an excitatory mechanism which exaggerates the effect of sensory input. There is a continuous barrage of activity from incoming nerve fibers on the spinal cord in the absence of stimulation and this is carried mainly in small fibers. Stimulation of higher centers can activate descending efferent fibers which influence conduction at spinal cord synapses; this mechanism provides a convenient explanation for the effect of central nervous system effects such as emotion and conditioning on pain.

How the gate works

The gate is normally kept open by tonic activity in small fibers which continues even in the absence of a noxious stimulus. This keeps the system in a state of readiness but it is easy to see how pain could be produced without noxious stimulation or disease, for example by the influence of central factors such as anxiety or depression on the gate.

Large and small fibers act on the T cells but also send communicating branches to the substantia gelatinosa cells, those from the large fibers being excitatory, those from the small fibers inhibitory. The cells of the substantia gelatinosa inhibit the efferent fiber terminals on the T cells; this inhibition is increased by activity in large fibers and decreased by activity in small fibers. The final discharge of the T cells is therefore controlled by the relative activity in large and small fibers. If a stimulus activates mainly large fibers, it will fire T cells and cause pain but also partially close the gate by increasing the inhibitory activity of the substantia gelatinosa cells on the T cell, cutting short the T cell discharge and the pain. It is thought that maneuvers such as vibration, rubbing and scratching may increase large fiber discharge and thereby diminish pain.

The firing of T cells, when it reaches a critical threshold, is believed to activate an action system which includes the sensory awareness of pain as well as rubbing and scratching, avoidance behavior such as withdrawal, and various reflex phenomena such as crying out, turning of the head and eyes to inspect the damage and autonomic reactions such as those of fight and flight.

Evidence for and against the gate
Evidence in support of the theory comes from electrical stimulation of nerves and from observation in post-herpetic neuralgia. Wall and Sweet (1967) found that threshold stimulation of peripheral nerves, which is assumed to activate only large fibers, abolished the ability of local pressure to cause pain. This is interpreted as 'gate closure' by reducing the effectiveness of afferent impulses on T cells and it offers a method by which control of various otherwise intractable pains might be achieved. Noordenbos (1968) studied nerves from patients after infection with *Herpes zoster* and found a dis-proportionate loss of large fibers; this leaves the unopposed action of small fibers on T cells, a wide open gate, and pain which may be caused by non-noxious stimuli such as light touch. The theory has been questioned by Schmidt (1972) and Iggo (1972) who point to conflicting evidence concerning the effects of small fiber stimulation on dorsal root potentials and question the evidence for continuous afferent small fiber activity. The gate theory remains a useful working hypothesis and provides an anatomical framework within which modifica-tion of stimuli by central and peripheral factors could explain the variability of the sensation we know as pain.

The mechanism of pain: psychological considerations

PERCEPTION AND REACTION

Marshall (1894) and Strong (1895) were the first to make a distinction between two components of pain, perception and reaction. Pain is not produced simply by a stimulus sufficiently noxious to activate the pain receptor and send a message on its way to the sensory cortex, a process which may be called the perception component of pain. The modification which this message undergoes so that its effect—the sensation of pain, which is not necessarily proportional to the stimulus—is termed the reaction component. Beecher (1962) advanced the following evidence in favor of the existence of the reaction component.

1. Great wounds may be painless and small wounds painful. Guthrie (1827) noted this in the Peninsular War and Beecher (1946) in the Second World War; it was a curious finding that patients with great wounds but no pain could still feel the effects of clumsy venepuncture, suggesting that the pain mechanism or perception component is intact and implying that it is the reaction to or interpretation of the noxious stimulus that has been modified. For perhaps the same reason, sportsmen become aware of their injury after the game.

2. Emotion, suggestion, hypnosis and placebo therapy can block pain and such block is presumably on the reaction component; one would not imagine for example that a placebo could affect the pain-producing mechanism or perception component in any way.

3. Lobotomy and sometimes drugs may make a patient comfortable even though he continues to be aware of pain and his pain mechanism is presumably intact; lobotomy has been regarded as a surgical lesion of the reaction component.

4. Beecher (1962) argues that narcotic analgesics are effective only when pain is judged significant; they have no effect on transient experimental pains which are without significance and in which the reaction component is presumably minimal; in other words narcotic analgesics also act on the reaction component of pain.

MECHANISMS OF PAIN

It is clear that pain does not depend simply on the peripheral stimulus, and experience in clinical medicine supports this view. Many clinical writers have noted that pain is not necessarily the result of local disease; Sir Benjamin Brodie (1837) for example, was consulted concerning a young lady with severe pain and tenderness of the knee which was not accompanied by local signs of disease; later the patient manifested other hysterical features. Brodie concluded that it was not uncommon for a joint to be painful so that it was thought to be the seat of some serious disease, although no such disease in reality existed. Devine and Merskey (1965) found that no less than 53 of 137 patients attending a general medical clinic with pain had no organic lesion to explain it. Pain may be produced in a number of ways and the scheme which follows is based on that of Hill (1970).

1. Pain may be caused by disease.

2. Pain may be normal; Trotter (1921) argues that though pain in disease serves no obviously useful purpose, it seems to have a protective function in normal people; absence of pain in congenital indifference to pain is a disadvantage and leads to severe trauma. Pain is an everyday experience which is felt in the same way as heat and cold, but not usually remembered.

3. Pain is sometimes caused by disorders of the pain-producing mechanism, for example by lesions of peripheral nerves or the thalamus.

4. Psychosomatic pain occurs when a painful physical disorder results from a psychological state, for example occipital muscle spasm in anxiety.

5. Psychogenic pain is the direct result of psychological disorders, such as anxiety and depression, which are common in patients whose pain cannot be explained by organic disease. Conversely pain is common in patients with such psychological disorders (Merskey and Spear, 1967). It is perhaps unfortunate that patients do not complain of psychogenic pain; Szasz (1957) emphasizes that the differentiation of organic and psychogenic pain is not based on any difference between the pains but on the judgement of the observer.

Pain, as seen in the medical clinic, is a complex pheno-menon of which the noxious stimulus is only a part; processing of the message plays a large part in determining the final sensation and it appears that pain may arise in the processing mechanism which may include the gate of Melzack and Wall (1965).

The measurement of experimental pain

PAIN THRESHOLD

Pain threshold is defined as "the first barely perceptible pain to appear in an instructed subject under given conditions of noxious stimulation" (Beecher, 1957). It is measured in terms of the stimulus as the lowest intensity which will cause pain. The perception of pain is usually revealed by a verbal statement and Beecher (1957) points out that it can therefore be measured only in conscious and co-operative man. Pain threshold is an experimental concept and opinion has held at one extreme that it is a physiological phenomenon akin to the electrical threshold of isolated nerve fibers, and at the other that it doesn't exist. The former view is untenable since it fails to take account of the processing which a noxious stimulus undergoes. That pain threshold is a valid measurement is supported firstly by the reasonable constancy of pain threshold in an individual which distinguishes him from others, and secondly by the relationships shown between pain threshold and various aspects of pathological pain (Keele, 1968; Huskisson and Hart, 1972). Though Hardy, Woolf and Goodell (1940), using themselves as subjects, found a remarkable constancy of pain threshold, Chapman and Jones (1944) using the same method in 200 subjects, found much wider variations and later authors agree. There is strikingly more variation between subjects than between different measurements in the same subject (Gaensler, 1951) suggesting that pain threshold is a distinct individual characteristic. Seevers and Pfeiffer (1936) using von Frey hairs, showed wide individual variation in pain threshold and though measurements were fairly constant over the course of hours, there was much greater variation from week to week. Many external factors vary from week to week and one would expect these variations to be reflected in the processing of pain.

THE IDEAL METHOD
OF MEASURING PAIN THRESHOLD

A wide variety of experimental procedures has been used to produce pain in man either to study the phenomenon or to measure the effects of drugs upon it. Hardy *et al.* (1952) suggested six requirements of an adequate method of measuring pain threshold:

1. Measurability of stimulus with reproducibility,
2. Controllability,
3. Adequate range from threshold to ceiling,
4. Production of minimal damage to tissue,
5. Convenience,
6. Production of clear-cut perception of pain.

Beecher (1957) adds:

7. Applicability to a body part where neuro-histological factors are at a minimum,
8. Possibility of carrying out repeated stimulation without interfering with subsequent determinations,
9. Sensitivity to analgesics.

Mechanical methods

Mechanical methods of producing pain have often been used because they are simple and acceptable to patients. Von Frey pressed horse hairs of various sizes on the skin and measured the hardness of the hair required to produce pain; this method was used by Seevers and Pfeiffer (1936) to test analgesics. Libman (1934) pressed on the styloid process with his thumb and graded the response; Pelner (1941) tried to eliminate the variability of the pressure applied by using a mechanical gauge pressed on the proximal phalanx of the thumb until it became unbearable. Hollander (1939) used a cheese grater concealed inside a sphygmomanometer cuff, which was inflated until the patient winced, changed expression or cried out. Algometers have apparently been used since Victorian times; McDougall used one to measure the pain threshold of Polynesians in 1903 (Merskey and Spear, 1969). More recently the method has been used by Hardy *et al.* (1952) who called it a coiled spring esthesiometer, Keele (1954), Clutton Brock (1964) and Huskisson and Hart (1972). The apparatus described by Keele (1954) consisted of a blunt-ended rod, one end of which was applied to the forehead of the patient. The other end was attached to a coiled spring; a scale measured the displacement of the rod and could be calibrated in kilograms. The pressure was increased at the rate of 1 kg per second and the end-point taken as the verbal statement of pain. Burn (1968) used a device which delivered a measurable blow to the soft tissues in front of the Achilles tendon, a site favored by clinicians for testing deep pain sensation.

Heat and cold
Extremes of heat and cold are painful and both have been used as noxious stimuli to produce experimental pain. Hardy *et al.* (1940) used radiant heat focused onto an area of blackened skin. A projection lamp is used as the heat source and a shutter exposes the subject to the stimulus for 3 seconds. The intensity of the stimulus can be raised and when the threshold is found, a measurement is made by introducing a radiometer into the path of the beam. Problems with the method, reviewed by Beecher (1957) include variations in blackness of the skin, changes in ambient temperature, effects of repeated stimulation particularly if there is tissue damage and technical problems such as changes in exposure time. Using this method, Hardy *et al.* (1952) produced a 'dol' scale of pain; they found that there were 21 just noticeable differences in intensity of pain between pain threshold and ceiling pain and called two such differences a dol. A modification of the method by D'Amour and Smith (1941) used a fixed intensity of heat and measured the time taken to produce pain. The method has been used in man by Lee and Pfeiffer (1951) who called their apparatus a warm-wire algesimeter and in animals by Woolfe and MacDonald (1944) who placed mice on a hot plate and measured the time taken to react. Wolff *et al.* (1969) used a modification of the cold pressor technique; the subject's hand was immersed in warm water then transferred to ice-water. Two end-points were measured, the subjects being asked to shout 'pain' when pain was felt and 'stop' when it became unbearable.

Electricity
The ease of controlling an electrical stimulus has contributed

to the popularity of this method of producing pain, which was first used by von Helmholtz in 1851 (Beecher, 1959). Later workers have applied electrical currents either to the skin or tooth pulp. The latter may have advantages over skin because it is less subject to external influences such as temperature and sweating. Brief shocks are applied to an amalgam filling in a tooth and threshold for pain determined. Because it is not possible to apply the method to a standard size filling in a standard position in a tooth, it is doubtful whether the method can be used to measure the pain threshold of an individual, though it has been used to follow changes after drug administration.

Vascular occlusion
Lewis *et al.* (1931) used a tourniquet applied to the upper arm in a patient who was contracting his hand muscles at a constant rate and measured the time taken to produce pain as the pain threshold. Hewer and Keele (1948) and later Smith and Beecher (1969) used the method to test analgesics.

Visceral and chemical methods
Methods of producing visceral pain are of great interest though their application is limited to very special situations such as surgical operations and the rather unusual volunteers found in American prisons. Gaensler (1951) distended the bile duct through a T tube and determined pain threshold. Chapman and Jones (1944) distended the esophagus by inflating a balloon introduced through the nose, the end-point being taken as a feeling of substernal fullness rather than pain. They were not able to produce a severe pain by this method, but pain threshold correlated with measurements using radiant heat. Lim and Guzman (1968) infused bradykinin into the peritoneum of volunteers, finding an optimum individual dose which caused pain. Armstrong *et al.* (1951) found that the concentration of pain-producing substances required to produce a certain intensity of pain was constant for a given individual and this is a measure of pain threshold.

End-points
Considerable confusion exists over the definition of end-points

in pain threshold studies. There are three quantities involved, pain threshold, severe pain threshold or pain reaction threshold, and pain tolerance.

If the intensity of a noxious stimulus is slowly increased, a point is reached at which pain is felt and this is the pain threshold. Because the patient is required to make a statement to this effect, Keele (1968) preferred to call it pain complaint threshold and other suggested terms include verbal report of pain (Hall and Stride, 1954), pain perception threshold (Merskey et al., 1962; Chapman and Jones, 1944; Gelfand et al., 1963) and lower pain threshold (Sternbach and Tursky, 1965).

If the intensity of the noxious stimulus continues to be increased after pain has been felt, another point is reached at which the patient says that the pain has become severe or 'hurts a lot' and this may be called the severe pain threshold (Merskey et al., 1962). Some authors have taken this point as intolerable pain which causes confusion with pain tolerance, discussed below. Others have taken some reaction to pain as the end-point; this may be wincing, withdrawal (Chapman and Jones, 1944) or changes in pulse rate (Hazouri and Mueller, 1950), and is appropriately called the pain reaction threshold. Sternbach and Tursky (1965) called it upper pain threshold.

Pain tolerance, expressed as usual with experimental pain in terms of the stimulus, is the difference between pain threshold and severe pain threshold or pain reaction threshold; it is therefore the quantity of pain-producing stimulus which can be tolerated. Gelfand et al. (1963) used an ultrasonic generator to apply heat to the thumb and measured pain threshold as the time after application when pain was first perceived. The subject was then asked to keep his thumb in contact with the painful stimulus until pain became unbearable; the difference in seconds between this point and pain threshold was called pain tolerance. It is not surprising that there was a good correlation between pain threshold and pain reaction threshold, the point of withdrawal of the thumb; this is a statistical artifact arising because pain threshold is a major component of pain reaction threshold. There was no significant correlation between pain threshold and pain tolerance. Merskey and Spear (1964), whose findings were the same, called pain tolerance the reaction interval; Wolff (1968) and Wolff *et al.* (1969) called it pain sensitivity range.

It is clear that different end-points will give different results and it follows that the end-point in any study of experimental pain must be carefully defined.

FACTORS AFFECTING EXPERIMENTAL PAIN

Beecher (1959) lists 27 different types of factor, other than analgesics which are said to produce variation in the pain threshold in man or animals. The following appear to be important in experimental pain in man and may be relevant to pathological pain.

Race

Pain has been found to be perceived at a lower level in negroes and people from Mediterranean countries (Chapman and Jones, 1944). Zborowski (1952) interviewed Americans of different racial origin and found differences in attitudes to pain and pain relief; Italians for example expressed a particular desire for pain relief. Sternbach and Tursky (1965) supported his findings in an experimental study using electrical stimulation in the same racial groups. Severe pain threshold was significantly lower in Italians though the difference in pain threshold was not significant.

Sex

Many studies have shown a lower pain threshold in women, including Wilder (1940) using the Hollander (1939) method, Sherman (1943) using the Libman (1934) and Hollander (1939) methods, Hall and Stride (1954) using radiant heat, Kennard (1959) using electrical stimulation, Dundee and Moore (1960) and Merskey and Spear (1964) using the algometer. Others who have not shown this difference include Hardy *et al.* (1952) and Chapman and Jones (1944) using radiant heat, and Huskisson and Hart (1972) using the algometer.

Age

Pain threshold has been found by several authors to rise with age (Chapman and Jones, 1944; Hall and Stride, 1954; Huskisson and Hart, 1972).

Skin temperature
Both mechanical and radiant heat methods of measuring pain threshold are affected by skin temperature. Hardy *et al.* (1952) showed a linear relationship using their radiant heat method. Wells (1947) used a spring clamp applied to his own finger and reported that local warmth up to 37 °C reduced the pain.

Tissue damage disease; nerve lesions
Tissue damage including skin lesions at the site of measurement of pain threshold increases sensitivity to pain (Hardy *et al.*, 1952). This may explain the tendency for measurements of pain threshold to fall with repetition (Merskey *et al.*, 1962). Pain threshold should not be confused with tenderness: pressure on an inflamed joint enables the observer to measure tenderness; pain threshold must not be measured in an area of disease since the disease severity will presumably contribute to the severity of pain. It is not surprising that pain threshold is elevated in areas of skin supplied by damaged nerves (Noter-mans, 1967).

Fatigue
Chapman and Jones (1944) found that whereas physical fatigue had no effect, mental fatigue lowered pain threshold in some subjects.

Fear of pain; anxiety
Pain threshold is lowered by fear of pain and anxiety. Under such conditions, Hill *et al.* (1952) found that subjects over-estimated the intensity of painful stimuli. Morphine reduced the anxiety and abolished the effect. In the absence of anxiety morphine had no effect on the ability to estimate pain severity.

Suggestion and attitudes of subject and observer
Elevation of pain threshold can be produced by hypnotic suggestion (Hardy *et al.*, 1952) and suggestion is widely used by doctors to improve the performance of the treatment they give! Pain threshold is likely to be influenced by the observer's explanation of his intentions and the subject's interpretation of them. The use of trained subjects has been advocated by some authors but there are disadvantages, in particular the

ability of trained observers to recognize drug effects other than by relief of pain. Beecher (1959) preferred subjects "who know nothing of the purpose of the experiment or the parameters at issue, and who care nothing about the outcome".

Distraction; pain elsewhere
Distraction of the subject by external events, such as noise, raises the pain threshold (Hardy *et al.*, 1952). Hippocrates observed that "of simultaneous pain in two places, the lesser is obliterated by the greater". This was confirmed experimentally by Hardy *et al.* (1940).

Placebo
A subject given a treatment which he believes to be analgesic will produce a greater elevation of pain threshold than another subject given the same treatment but not expecting pain relief. Gelfand *et al.* (1963) showed statistically significant differences between the effects of placebo combined with anticipation and no treatment on both pain threshold and pain tolerance.

Side effects of drugs
Some effects of drugs other than the production of analgesia may alter pain threshold. They include nausea, which lowers pain threshold and interferes with analgesics, peripheral vasoconstriction, respiratory depression and carbon dioxide retention, and impaired judgement which interferes with the recognition and reporting of pain threshold.

Laterality
Wolff and Jarvik (1964) showed that pain perception may vary on the dominant and non-dominant sides of the body. Using cold to produce pain, they showed that measurements using the right or dominant hand showed better correlations with other methods of measuring pain threshold than the left or non-dominant hand. This suggests that the left or non-dominant side of the body is less well developed for pain sensation in a way analogous to motor precision. It is of interest that some authors have found psychogenic pain to be commoner on the left side (Edmonds, 1947). Huskisson (1973) failed to confirm these observations using the Hollander (1939)

method and the algometer method described by Keele (1948). The results are shown in Table 1.1. There was an equally good correlation between pain threshold measured by algometer and the Hollander method using the left and right arms, and mean pain threshold in the two arms was almost exactly the same. Large differences appeared when the group was divided according to the order of performance of the test, the second arm tested giving lower results.

Table 1.1 EFFECTS OF LATERALITY AND ORDER OF TESTING ON PAIN THRESHOLD MEASURED BY HOLLANDER (1939) METHOD. CORRELATION COEFFICIENTS WITH PAIN THRESHOLD MEASURED BY ALGOMETER AND MEAN LEVELS BY BOTH METHODS ARE SHOWN

Arm tested	Number of subjects	Order of testing	Mean pain threshold		Correlation coefficient
			Hollander	Algometer	
R	25 25	{ R before L { L before R	88.5	3.4	0.55
L	25 25	{ R before L { L before R	88.9	3.4	0.56
R	25	R before L	99.4	3.2	0.58
R	25	L before R	77.6	3.5	0.62
L	25	R before L	76.1	3.2	0.61
L	25	L before R	101.7	3.5	0.52

Personality

Gelfand *et al.* (1963) showed a significant correlation between pain tolerance and measures of poise, ascendancy and self-assurance, using the California personality inventory. There was no correlation between pain threshold and any personality trait. Collins (1965) found that both pain threshold and severe pain threshold were related to childhood protection; there was an inverse relationship with childhood independence. It was surmised that increased experience of pain in childhood results in greater sensitivity to pain.

Analgesics and pain threshold

It is disappointing that despite considerable effort, no accepted method exists for the evaluation of analgesics in normal subjects using experimental pain. Different studies have produced conflicting results and in many some or all of the subjects studied have failed to show elevation of pain threshold in response even to narcotic analgesics. Another problem is that drugs which are not accepted as analgesic in pathological pain may affect experimental pain, for example barbiturates, which were found to be more effective than aspirin or codeine in raising the threshold to electrical stimulation of the skin (Wolff *et al.*, 1969), and adrenalin, which affects the threshold as determined by tooth pulp stimulation (Ivy *et al.*, 1962). Houde *et al.* (1948) reported a patient in whom an analgesic produced a large elevation of pain threshold though his pain recurred while the threshold was elevated. Hardy *et al.* (1940) showed that the pain-threshold elevating effect of morphine was abolished by the production of experimental pain at another site, and Hewer and Keele (1948) interpreted this as indicating that analgesics were acting on the reaction component of, pain. If this were so, one might expect the peripherally acting analgesics such as aspirin to have an effect on pain threshold, but the response to them has been no more consistent than that to morphine-like drugs.

Four exceptions seem to exist to the conclusion that elevation of pain threshold is not a feature of the analgesic effects of drugs. Firstly experimental methods in animals such as the tail-flick method have been useful in testing analgesics. Secondly dental pulp stimulation has proved useful in some studies in man. Thirdly it appears that the closer experimental pain becomes to pathological pain, the more likely it is that it will be affected by analgesics. Fourthly there is evidence that pain tolerance rather than threshold is improved by analgesics.

Hattemer *et al.* (1972) have been able to produce dose-response curves for aspirin using experimental dental pain. Goldberg and Huldt (1972) used the method successfully to show the effects of pentazocine (which is not effective in animal tests such as the tail-flick or mouse hot-plate methods), oral codeine and pethidine but not placebo. Kryger and Aggerbeck (1968) were able to demonstrate the prolonged effectiveness of a new formulation of dextro-propoxyphene.

Gaensler (1951) was able to demonstrate the effects of narcotic analgesics but not aspirin or placebo on pain induced by biliary distension which resembles pathological pain. Lim and Guzman (1968) found oral aspirin effective for pain induced by intraperitoneal bradykinin.

Wolff *et al.* (1969), using cold-induced pain to measure pain threshold and tolerance (the difference between threshold and intolerable pain which they called pain sensitivity range), found that analgesics caused little change in pain threshold though there were big differences in pain tolerance. Smith and

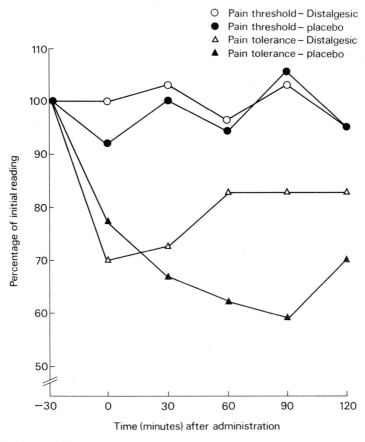

Figure 1.1   Effects of an analgesic (Distalgesic) and placebo on pain threshold and pain tolerance. Distalgesic or identical placebo tablets were administered at time 0. Differences in pain threshold were not statistically significant; pain tolerance was significantly higher after Distalgesic than placebo. Distalgesic is a combination analgesic containing dextropropoxyphene 32.5 mg and paracetamol (acetaminophen) 325 mg.

Beecher (1969) used a modification of the tourniquet method and measured the time taken to produce various grades from the threshold to unbearable pain. Aspirin had no effect on pain threshold, slight pain or unbearable pain; however there was a significant reduction in the time taken to cause moderately distressing or very distressing pain. This accords with experience that aspirin has no effect on agonizing or unbearable pain, which requires narcotics (Hill and Turner, 1969), relieves intermediate grades of pain and has no effect on pain threshold. Huskisson (1973) used the Hollander (1939) method to measure pain threshold and tolerance, the difference in mmHg between the threshold and the level which caused intolerable pain. The results are shown in Figure 1.1; threshold was unaffected but the fall in pain tolerance was less after an analgesic than placebo.

Effect of pain threshold on response to analgesics
Patients with a low pain threshold are more likely to respond to analgesics; Dundee and Moore (1960) showed a more consistent response to pethidine in post-operative patients with low pain threshold and pain reaction thresholds, measured by an algometer designed by Clutton-Brock (1964). Gaensler (1951) studied the rise in pain threshold measured by bile duct distension, in patients given narcotic analgesics; a greater rise occurred in those with initially low thresholds. This is probably explained by the greater pain severity in patients with low pain threshold (see below).

Gelfand *et al.* (1963) found that patients with low pain threshold also responded better to placebo than those with high pain thresholds; they used an ultrasonic apparatus applied to the thumb to produce deep heat and pain. On the other hand, a high tolerance was associated with large changes in response to placebo.

PAIN THRESHOLD IN DISEASE
Several groups of workers have found low pain thresholds in patients with neuroses. Sherman (1943) compared pain threshold in patients with organic and functional disease, using the Libman (1934) and Hollander (1939) methods; pain threshold was higher in those with organic disease. Wilder

(1940) used the Hollander (1939) method and results were similar. Chapman *et al.* (1947) used the radiant heat method to study patients with psychoneuroses; whereas pain threshold was normal, pain reaction threshold, judged by wincing, was low and patients with psychoneuroses also showed a more pronounced motor withdrawal. Hall and Stride (1944) using the same method found that anxiety neurotics both perceived and reacted to pain earlier than depressed patients; successful electro-convulsive therapy for depression was associated with a significant lowering of pain threshold. Smith (1967), using the algometer described by Keele (1954), found lower pain thresholds in patients who frequently attended a general practitioner's surgery than in a normal control population; pain threshold was also lower in those who were emotionally disturbed or complained of pain without a demonstrable organic basis.

Since pain threshold is raised by the production of experimental pain at another site, high levels might be expected in patients with painful diseases. There is little evidence to support this though Huskisson and Hart (1972), using the algometer, found high levels in patients with ankylosing spondylitis, and Hazouri and Mueller (1950), using radiant heat, reported three patients with intractable pain, in whom relief of pain by spino-thalamic tractotomy was associated with a fall in pain threshold. They also found that pain threshold in paraplegics with pain did not differ from normal and other studies in painful states agree. Kennard (1959) using electrical stimulation, showed no difference in pain threshold between a group of patients with chronic severe pain and a control group; Hardy and Javert (1949) using radiant heat found normal pain thresholds in women in labor; Huskisson and Hart (1972) using the algometer, found normal levels in rheumatoid arthritis and Dundee and Moore (1960) found low levels in post-operative patients with skin incisions.

Keele (1968) used the algometer to study pain threshold in patients with myocardial infarction. He showed that pain threshold was inversely related to the severity, duration and extent of radiation of pain and to the analgesic dosage required to relieve pain. Patients with low pain thresholds had more severe pain which lasted for longer and spread over larger areas of the body; they required more doses of morphine for relief of pain during their illness. Disease severity, as judged by peak enzyme levels and the extent of electrocardiographic changes, was also related to both pain and morphine requirements. Huskisson and Hart (1972), using the same method in patients with rheumatoid arthritis, also found pain threshold inversely related to severity and duration of pain and to analgesic requirements. The same authors showed that pain threshold and disease severity were of about equal importance in determining the severity of pain, and that these two factors accounted for a large part of the variation in pain severity (Huskisson and Hart, 1971). A number of observations have suggested that patients with rheumatoid arthritis and a high pain threshold might be liable to develop more severe joint damage because they are able to remain mobile and may therefore continue unsuitable work. This assumes a protective function for pathological pain; in support Bywaters (1964) found cystic changes in x-rays of the hands of patients with little pain, strong muscles and heavy jobs who continued to work despite their arthritis. Castillo et al. (1965) showed an inverse relation between radiological articular erosions and porosis; heavy manual work was associated with larger erosions and less porosis and Scott (1965) suggested that this might be related to the pain threshold of the patient. Rest has a favorable effect on the symptoms of the disease, at least for a time, and denervation of a limb protects against rheumatoid arthritis (Kamerman, 1966; Glick, 1967). However Huskisson and Hart (1972) found no relationship between pain threshold and progression of disease or radiological changes and no evidence that patients with low pain threshold fared better than their more stoical comrades. In agreement with this, Clark (1951) reported a patient with rheumatoid arthritis and congenital indifference to pain in whom the association appeared to be beneficial, and de Haas (1972) described a series of cases of rheumatoid arthritis which he called 'typus robustus'. Despite active arthritis and unfavorable prognostic features, these patients remained at work, had little pain and did not apparently develop progressive joint destruction.

A high pain threshold is an advantage, making disease less painful and analgesics less necessary; it follows that pain in disease is a disadvantage. There is no evidence that a high pain threshold predisposes to traumatic changes in the presence of disease, as congenital indifference to pain does in its absence. There is therefore no reason why measures should not be taken to raise pain threshold. Huskisson and Hart (1972) suggested that the high pain threshold found in ankylosing spondylitis might be due to the attitude to the disease, patients being encouraged to lead normal lives which they usually achieve. Confirmation of this must await a prospective study but in the meantime, there is no harm in encouraging patients with chronic painful disease to lead active and fulfilling lives.

Measurement of pain in disease

AVAILABLE METHODS

Though some efforts have been made to evaluate the effectiveness of treatment for several centuries (Green, 1954), it is only in the last 30 years that formal measurement of pain severity has been attempted and used for the clinical trial of substances with analgesic properties. Many of the methods used are borrowed from psychology. Freyd (1921) listed ways in which such quantities could be rated; those applicable to pain or pain relief can be summarized as follows:

(1) *The quantal method* in which pain is either present or absent, or a defined level of pain relief is attained.

(2) *Numerical or descriptive rating scales*, in which pain is graded in severity by numbers, for example 1 to 5 or by descriptions such as mild and severe.

(3) *Percentage and fraction methods*; assuming that the maximum possible pain or pain at a particular time such as the start of an experiment is 100% or 1, subsequent experience can be rated either as a percentage or a fraction of the reference level.

(4) *Ranking methods* in which pain on different occasions is said to be better or worse, or different treatments placed in order of pain-relieving activity. Preference is often used to determine order of effectiveness.

(5) *Visual analogue scales*, representing pain as a straight line, the extremes of which are defined as the extremes of pain.

(6) *The graphic rating method* in which descriptive phrases are distributed in order of severity along the straight line of a visual analogue scale.

Quantal method

The earliest work used the quantal method and measured the number of subjects achieving complete pain relief either in post-operative pain or pain due to cancer (Lee, 1942). Different doses of intra-muscular morphine were used, increasing until either complete pain relief occurred or it became evident that this would not occur at a reasonable dose; the average effective dose was found to be 9.6 mg. The decision about therapeutic effectiveness was made by nurses and physicians. This technique was extended with a much more sophisticated design by Denton and Beecher (1949). They used placebo and standard reference drugs as well as an unknown compound in crossover studies, randomizing the order of administration. Relief of pain in post-operative patients was graded as none, slight, moderate or complete; moderate or complete relief was taken as significant and stated to be at least 50% relief of pain; again this judgement was made by professional observers, trained experienced technicians or nurses. 82% of patients had significant pain relief with 4–6 mg of morphine per 150 pounds body weight, rising to 93% with 7–9 mg, with no further increase thereafter. The same technique was used in a later study of the effectiveness of aspirin and oral narcotic drugs, again in post-operative pain (Beecher, Keats, Mosteller and Lasagna, 1953). Among placebo reactors there was little or no difference between percentages relieved by different drugs but elimination of placebo reactors improved the results showing aspirin 600 mg superior to oral morphine or codeine. Significant pain relief was attained after 25%–40% of doses of placebo compared to 50% of doses of aspirin 300 mg (difference not statistically significant) and 55% of doses of aspirin 600 mg (statistically highly significant). This study can be criticized on the grounds that repeated doses of alternate treatments were given to the same patient every two hours, not long enough apart to eliminate additive effects. The results are somewhat unconvincing because the lowest percentage of pain relief with placebo occurred in the experiment with high dose aspirin accentuating a very small difference. Beecher (1957), reviewing this work, emphasized the desirability of crossover studies, using the patient as his own control, the used of paired comparisons, testing drug and placebo under comparable circumstances and the double-blind technique to eliminate bias on the part of both subject and observer.

Descriptive rating scale
Beecher's work was directed at finding compounds which produced significant pain relief (arbitrarily defined) within a significant period of time and for a minimum period of time. Other workers have sought to improve the sensitivity of measurement by using quantitative methods rather than the quantal method. Keele (1948) defined pain in five grades, none, slight (awareness of pain without distress), moderate (distracts attention from a routine occupation such as reading or housework), severe (fills the field of consciousness to the exclusion of other events and often has visceral accompaniments), and agonizing (accompanied by motor effects such as restlessness). He found patients able to record their pain severity and in a later study used the method to demonstrate the effect of morphine (Hewer *et al.*, 1949). Houde *et al.* (1960) used the same pain severity scale, recording changes hourly for six hours after administration of drugs in patients with chronic pain due to malignant disease. Measurements were made by a trained nurse. They used crossover designs and controlled their experiments with placebo and reference standards. A curve of pain severity against time after drug administration was obtained; the area under the curve was used to provide a total relief score. A simple pain scale, as described by Keele (1948) but omitting agonizing pain, has been used successfully by Huskisson *et al.* (1970) to demonstrate the analgesic properties of aspirin and Ibuprofen in rheumatoid arthritis. In the same study, a nine point scale of change was used, giving an increase in sensitivity over the four-point pain scale.

Percentage method
Copeman (1950) used percentage method to record pain. The patient started at 100% and moved up or down according to progress. Huskisson *et al.* (1969) used this method to measure the effects of analgesics but Hart and Huskisson (1972) criticized it because the scale had no descriptive limits; one patient might score moderate relief of pain as 80%, another as 20%. A fraction method has been used for pain relief (Swerdlow *et al.*, 1963)

Preference

Preference is widely used in drug studies though Hart and Huskisson (1972) pointed out that it was composed of many factors and might therefore be misleading. For example Huskisson (1973) noted in a single-dose analgesic study that patients sometimes preferred a drug which produced less pain relief because it was free of side effects. Huskisson and Grayson (1974) noted that preference could be an oversimplification of a therapeutic response. In a trial of a hypnotic and an analgesic, preferences showed a trend which was not statistically significant. Analysis of two separate components of the response, relief of pain and improved sleep, suggested that the trend was due to improvement in one but not the other. It is certainly not possible to equate preference and analgesia.

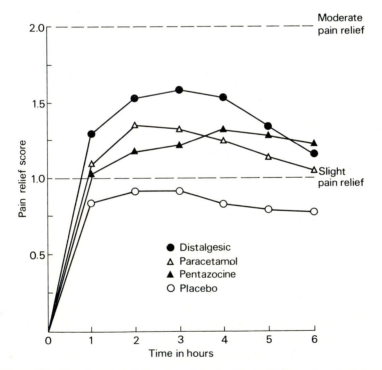

Figure 1.2   Use of a pain relief score to show the effects of three oral analgesics and placebo in rheumatoid arthritis. Two tablets of each were given. Paracetamol tablets contained 500 mg and pentazocine 25 mg.

Pain relief scales

When pain is measured after the administration of an analgesic, pain relief at a particular time is calculated by subtracting the pain score from the initial pain severity. Unless all patients have the same initial pain severity, it is necessary to assume that reduction of pain from severe to moderate is the same as reduction from moderate to slight and slight to none. A patient who receives an analgesic for slight pain has only one possible grade of improvement which is complete relief of pain; this is unusual especially with simple analgesics such as aspirin which relieve but do not abolish pain. This problem can be partly overcome by using pain relief scores so that all patients start from the same point, and all have the same number of possible grades of improvement. This method has been criticized on the grounds that the patient must remember his initial pain severity (Parkhouse and Holmes, 1963) and for this reason, such a scale would be unsuitable for studies lasting for long periods of time. On the other hand, it is more usual for a patient to express himself in this way; he says "my pain is slightly better" rather than "my pain is now only moderately severe". Pain relief scales have been used by Dundee (1960) who scored analgesia as excellent, good, moderate, poor and doubtful or absent; Swerdlow *et al.* used a four point scale: pain unabated, less than half relieved, more than half relieved and completely relieved. This scale could be extended by using smaller fractions. Huskisson (1973) used a pain relief scale to measure the effects of single doses of analgesics in rheumatoid arthritis; an example is shown in Figure 1.2.

Visual analogue scale

A visual analogue scale is a line whose boundaries are defined as the extremes of the quantity to be measured. With this method, subjective states can be assessed on a continuous scale between the defined limits (Figure 1.3).

Between the limits of agonizing pain and no pain on Keele's (1948) scale, there are only three single points, severe, moderate and mild, and few intermediate descriptive terms are available. The relative sizes of differences between descriptive terms are unknown and the assumption must be made when attaching scores to them, that the differences between each point are

Pain as bad as it could be

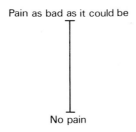

No pain

Figure 1.3 Visual analogue pain scale. The patient is asked to mark the line at a point corresponding to his pain severity

equal. The visual analogue scale introduces an infinite number of points between the extremes of the scale. These scales were popular at the beginning of the century and are enjoying a revival. Aitken (1969) stressed the advantage of sensitivity in the use of visual analogue scales; he found reasonable correlations with other methods of measuring the same quantity and satisfactory consistency between repeated measurements. He quotes the application of the method to a variety of subjective states including depression, alertness, quality of sleep, dyspnea and dyspepsia. Clark and Spear (1964) used a visual analogue scale to measure well-being and concluded that it was both reliable and sensitive; it is difficult to define reliability in terms of repeated measurements of subjective states since pain especially is not expected to remain the same even from one minute to the next. Bond and Pilowsky (1966) used a visual analogue scale to measure pain, defining the extremes as "I have no pain at all" and "My pain is as bad as it could possibly be". Berry and Huskisson (1973) found a good correlation between the results of a visual analogue scale and a simple descriptive pain scale and the mean points corresponding to his descriptive terms—mild, moderate and severe—were spaced out evenly along the line. They argued that calibration of the visual analogue scale in this way increased the descriptive value of the results since a reduction of mean pain from moderate to mild has more meaning to a clinician than a set of figures taken from a visual analogue scale.

THE GRAPHIC RATING METHOD

It is a logical step from the findings of Berry and Huskisson (1973), to suggest the use of a visual analogue scale with 'calibrations', descriptive terms or guide words placed at suitable intervals along its length before the measurement is made. This has proved to have advantages and also disadvantages. Freyd (1921) used this method to measure psychological traits and based on his experience suggested the following rules for constructing a graphic rating scale:

(1) Define the trait to be rated.

(2) Decide on the extremes of the trait; the end phrases should not be so extremely worded as never to be employed.

(3) Introduce the scale with an appropriate question.

(4) Use a line of such length that a stencil can easily be calibrated and not too long so that it can be grasped as a unit.

(5) There should be no breaks or divisions in the line.

(6) There should be not more than 5 nor less than 3 descriptive terms; the phrase describing the average of the trait should be in the center of the scale. Only universally understood phrases should be used; they should be short and precise in meaning. There should be a clearly visible gap between each.

(7) The favorable extreme of the scale should be alternated.

Freyd (1921) noted the tendency for results to be concentrated over certain descriptive phrases leading to an uneven distribution of measurements; in one trait there was a concentration over the term 'agreeable' whereas no-one was rated 'grouchy and unpleasant'. The advantage of the method is that it enables the rater to make as fine a discrimination as he wishes while retaining the descriptive value of a simple rating scale. The distribution of results can be improved by varying the size of differences between terms, though as Freyd points out, we have no notion of the true distribution of such traits as good nature or self-esteem — nor of pain severity. Huskisson *et al.* (1973) used a graphic rating method (Figure 1.4) in a clinical trial of an analgesic for rheumatoid arthritis. The distribution of pain measurements is shown in Figure 1.5 and it is clear that the patients preferred the descriptive terms to

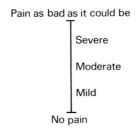

Figure 1.4 Graphic rating scale for pain

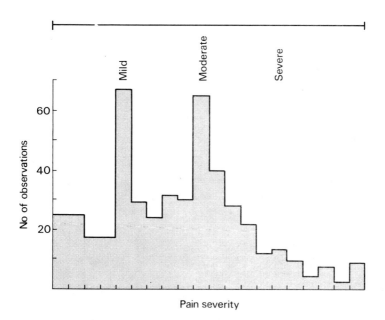

Figure 1.5 Distribution of results of measurement of pain severity, using the graphic rating method illustrated in Figure 1.4

the areas between. Though patients sometimes claim that their pain severity lies between the descriptive terms of a simple pain scale, it appears that most do not take advantage of the increased sensitivity offered by a graphic rating scale; in a separate experiment, Huskisson (1973) found that only 27% of patients used points between the descriptive terms of a graphic rating scale. It was our impression that patients preferred the graphic rating scale, finding it easier to understand, and in a formal comparison, Huskisson (1973) found 7% of patients unable to complete a visual analogue scale satisfactorily whereas only 4% were unable to complete a graphic rating scale.

Measurement by subject or observer

A number of groups have used a trained observer to measure pain. Lee (1942) tried to use questionnaires which the patients completed but failed because the patients were either apathetic if their pain was relieved, or if it was not, 'unreasonable' in exaggerating their discomfort. Pain charts completed by patients were abandoned by Houde *et al.* (1960) who found that they were not always completed regularly and suggested that introspection led to an undue influence of emotional factors. Parkhouse and Holmes (1963) also favored the use of an observer pointing out that some patients are known to exaggerate the severity of their pain. In an experiment designed to test the observer against the subject, they carried out a doubleblind trial of morphine and saline in post-operative patients. The number either improved or not improved was judged to be greater by the observer than by the subjects. The difference between morphine and saline was not statistically significant using the subject's opinion, a finding which is difficult to understand in view of the effectiveness of morphine demonstrated in many other studies. A simple descriptive rating scale was also used by patients and observers and again the differences between morphine and saline showed observer rating to be the more sensitive.

On the other hand Keele (1948) found that patients were able to record their pain severity on his descriptive rating scale and in almost all cases welcomed the task. This has also been our experience, and it is difficult to understand how an observer can decide the severity of pain, a completely subjective experience. Though this decision can only be made by the subject, an 'observer' may be helpful in ensuring that measurements are made at the appropriate times and in explaining the pain chart to him. It is certainly our experience that an experienced person is required to assist patients with visual analogue scales at their first and often subsequent use. Though Parkhouse and Holmes (1963) point out that patients exaggerate pain, it would be impossible to accept pain measurements in which the observer has decided, for example, that a patient who claims to have severe pain, has moderate pain and is exaggerating. In double-blind studies, the use of an observer provides an additional possible source of error; an experienced observer might recognize effects of drugs other than analgesia, for example, small pupils, drowsiness or euphoria after morphine. The observer is also liable to the error, mentioned by Merskey and Spear (1967), of confusing the stimulus with the experience. Would Beecher's soldiers with serious wounds have been accused of minimizing their pain? Pain is a personal psychological experience and an observer can play no legitimate part in its direct measurement.

Matching methods

Hardy, Woolf and Goodell (1956) suggested that pathological pain could be measured in dols by matching the severity of experimental pain, induced by heat, to that of pathological pain. Kast (1968) used the same principle and a machine, operated by the patient, which applied pressure to the fingertip. Good correlations were apparently achieved between pain measured thus and simultaneously measured by the patient, an observer and by observation of behavior signs of pain, all on a four-point rating scale. It must be difficult to match the severity of different types of pain, for instance pin-prick and biliary colic.

An alternative to verbal expression

Armstrong *et al.* (1953) used a mechanical method of recording pain as an alternative to verbal statement. The subjects squeezed a bag, increasing the tightness of squeezing in proportion to the severity of pain. The strength of grip was recorded on a kymograph so that the duration of the pain could also be measured. They obtained consistent results even with inexperienced subjects, judged by the response to repeated identical applications of chemicals to a blister base.

Behaviorist methods

In the methods described above, measurement of pain is based on the opinion of the subject, even if an observer uses it to record the result himself; these methods have been called 'introspective', while another group of methods in which measurement of pain is based on some response on the part of the subject, has been called 'behaviorist' (Parkhouse and Holmes, 1963).

Lim and Guzman (1968) investigated the objective manifestations of pain in man by taking videotape pictures of prison volunteers while infusing bradykinin into their peritoneal cavities. They concluded that objective manifestations were less reliable than verbal report of pain because man is able to control his behavior to a degree which depends on individual circumstances including personality, conditioning, training and past experience. 81% of their volunteers felt pain regularly with intraperitoneal bradykinin but only 52% showed facial signs interpreted as indicating pain, such as grimacing and only 31% continued to do this repeatedly with each infusion. Vocalization, a cry or a groan, was even less frequent. These phenomena cannot therefore be relied upon as indicators of pain; they will be absent in the 'stiff-upper-lipped' and not consistently present in others.

Attempts have been made to use measurement of respiratory function as a measure of pain after abdominal surgery. Masson (1962) showed that vital capacity was increased by morphine after major upper gastro-intestinal surgery and Parkhouse and Holmes (1963) found vital capacity as sensitive as an observer's rating of pain. Though apparently objective, Masson (1962) points out that the measurement reflects the amount of effort the patient is willing to expend.

Huskisson (1974) measured urinary catecholamine excretion in patients with pain and showed that this was reduced when pain was relieved. This method, though indirect, may provide a useful measure of pain in crossover experiments, but will also reflect other subjective responses such as anxiety.

FACTORS AFFECTING RELIEF OF PAIN

Pain relief is as complex as pain itself and the therapeutic effectiveness of a drug is not the only factor in determining its

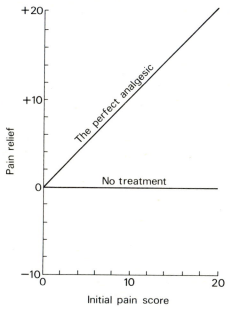

Figure 1.6   Theoretical relationship between pain relief and initial pain severity with no treatment and a hypothetical perfect analgesic

extent. Of particular importance are initial pain severity, the patient and his disease, the doctor, the therapeutic context, order of administration of drugs and side effects.

Initial pain severity
The theoretical relationship between initial pain severity and pain relief is shown in Figure 1.6; analgesics which are less than perfect lie between the perfect analgesic and no treatment. An example is shown in Figure 1.7; there is a striking relationship —patients with severe pain have an excellent chance of pain relief from analgesics whereas patients with mild pain need hardly bother to take them. Swerdlow *et al.* (1963) found narcotic analgesics more effective in patients with severe post-operative pain, while aspirin and compound codeine were more effective in slight pain.

There is some disagreement as to the effects of initial pain severity on placebo response. Beecher (1956) found placebo more effective on the first of four administrations to patients

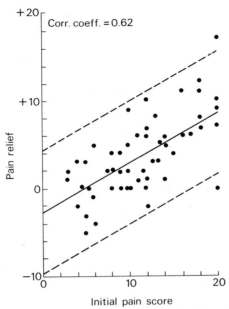

Figure 1.7 Relationship between pain relief and initial pain severity in patients with rheumatoid arthritis taking non-steroidal anti-inflammatory drugs

with post-operative pain and thought that this was because pain was more severe. Traut and Passarelli (1957) found placebo more effective in patients with severe rheumatoid arthritis. On the other hand Loan *et al.* (1968) found a placebo response less likely with severe initial pain and Dundee (1960) stated that very few patients with pain from intractable malignancy obtained relief from placebo tablets.

The patient and his disease
Lasagna (1964) emphasizes the need to consider population differences in analgesic studies. The significance of pain and its response to drugs may vary considerably in patients dying from cancer, recovering from operations, or living with arthritis. Batterman and Lower (1968) showed differences in the incidence of placebo response following active treatment in different races, sexes and diseases; in rheumatoid arthritis the combination of pain and inflammation may confuse interpretation of drug effects; steroids for example relieve pain without being analgesic.

The doctor—therapeutic context; order of treatment
Balint (1964) has written of the drug 'Doctor' and the effect he
has on the effectiveness of his prescription. Placebos are effective only in the therapeutic context of an active drug, analgesia
being induced by drugs given for pain, hypnosis for sleep, etc.
Similarly placebo is more effective given after an active drug
than before (Kantor *et al.*, 1966) and this effect is not abolished
by telling the patient that the treatment is different or by
making the treatments of different color (Huskisson, 1973).

Side effects
Effects of drugs other than those on the pain mechanism may
have a profound effect on pain; drugs which reduce spasm are
particularly effective in biliary colic; drugs which cause
unpleasant side effects such as nausea may be less effective in
relieving pain.

Present methods available for the relief of pain are
inadequate and one hopes that further exploration of the
mechanisms and factors which affect pain and its relief may
lead to better treatment of the unnecessary pain of disease and
better understanding of the normal pain of normal people.

REFERENCES

Aitken, R. C. B. (1969), *Proc. Roy. Soc. Med.*, *62*, 989

Armstrong, D., Dry, R. M. L., Keele, C. A. and Markham, J. W. (1951). *J. Physiol.* (Lond.), *115*, 59

Armstrong, D., Dry, R. M. L., Keele, C. A. and Markham, J. W. (1953). *J. Physiol.* (Lond.), *120*, 326

Balint, M. (1964). *The Doctor, his Patient and the Illness.* 2nd edition. London: Pitman

Batterman, R. C. and Lower, W. R. (1968). *Curr. Ther. Res.*, *10*, 136

Beecher, H. K. (1946). *Ann. Surg.*, *123*, 96

Beecher, H. K., Keats, A. S., Mosteller, F. and Lasagna, L. (1953). *J. Pharmacol.*, *109*, 393

Beecher, H. K. (1956). *Amer. J. Physiol.*, *187*, 163

Beecher, H. K. (1957). *Pharm. Rev.*, *9*, 59

Beecher, H. K. (1959). *Measurement of Subjective Responses.* New York: Oxford University Press

Beecher, H. K. (1962). In *The Assessment of Pain in Man and Animals.* Keele, C. A. and Smith, R. (editors). London: Livingstone

Berry, H. and Huskisson, E. C. (1972). *Clinical Trials Journal*, *9*, 13

Bishop, G. H. (1946). *Physiol. Rev.*, *26*, 77

Bond, M. R. and Pilowsky, I. (1966. *J. Psychosom. Res.*, *10*, 203

Brodie, B. B. (1837). *Lectures Illustrative of Certain Central Nervous System Affections, No. 2.*
    London: Longman
Burn, G. P. (1968). *Brit. J. Pharmacol. Chemotherap.*, *34*, 251
Bywaters, E. G. L. (1964). In *Radiological Aspects of Rheumatoid Arthritis*. Carter, M. E.
    (editor). Amsterdam. Excerpta Medica Foundation
Castillo, B. A., El Sallab, R. A. and Scott, J. T. (1965). *Ann. rheum. Dis.*, *24*, 522
Clutton Brock, J. (1964). *Anaesthesia*, *19*, 593
Chapman, W. P., Finesinger, J. E., Jones, C. M. and Cobb, S. (1947). *Arch. Neurol.
    Psychiat.*, *57*, 32
Chapman, W. P. and Jones, C. M. (1944). *J. Clin. Invest.*, *23*, 81
Clark, C. J. M. (1951). *Ann. rheum. Dis.*, *10*, 105
Clark, P. R. F. and Spear, F. G. (1964). *Bull. Brit. Psychol. Soc.*, *17*, 55
Collins, L. G. (1965). *Perceptual Motor Skills*, *21*, 349
Copeman, W. S. C. (1950). *Brit. med. J.*, *2*, 849
D'Amour, F. A. and Smith, D. L. (1941). *J. Pharmacol.*, *72*, 74
de Haas, W. H. D., de Boer, W., Griffioen, F. and Oosten-Elst, P. (1972). Paper
    presented at a combined meeting of the Heberden Society and the Dutch Society
    of Rheumatologists
Devine, R. and Merskey, H. (1965). *J. Psychosom. Res.*, *9*, 311
Douglas, W. W. and Ritchie, J. M. (1957). *J. Physiol. (Lond.)*, *139*, 385
Dundee, J. W. (1960). *Brit. J. Anaesth.*, *32*, 48
Dundee, J. W. and Moore, J. (1960). *Brit. J. Anaesth.*, *32*, 396
Edmonds, E. P. (1947). *Ann. rheum. Dis.*, *6*, 36
Ferreira, S. H. (1972). *Nature New Biology*, *240*, 200
Freyd, M. (1923). *J. educ. Psychol.*, *14*, 83
Gaensler, E. A. (1951). *J. Clin. Invest.*, *30*, 406
Gelfand, S., Ullman, L. P. and Krasner, L. (1963). *J. Nerv. Ment. Dis.*, *136*, 379
Glick, E. N. (1967). *Brit. med. J.*, *3*, 26
Goldberg, L. and Huldt, S. (1972). In *Pain*. Janzen, R., Keidel, W. D., Herz, A. and
    Steichele, C. (editors). London: Churchill Livingstone
Green, F. H. K. (1954). *Lancet, ii*, 1085
Guthrie, G. J. (1827). *A Treatise on Gunshot Wounds*. London: Burgess and Hill
Hall, K. R. L. and Stride, E. (1954). *Brit. J. Med. Psychol.*, *27*, 48
Hardy, J. D. and Javert, C. T. (1949). *J. Clin. Invest.*, *28*, 153
Hardy, J. D., Wolff, H. G. and Goodell, H. (1940). *J. Clin. Invest.*, *19*, 649
Hardy, J. D., Wolff, H. G. and Goodell, H. (1952). *Pain Sensations and Reactions.*
    Baltimore: Williams and Wilkins
Hattemer, H., Huber, H., Ziel, R. and Kunz, H. A. (1972). *Agents and Actions*, *2*, 176
Hazouri, L. A. and Mueller, A. D. (1950). *Arch. Neurol.*, *64*, 607
Hart, F. D. and Huskisson, E. C. (1972). *Lancet, i*, 28
Hensel, H., Iggo, A. and Witt, I. (1960). *J. Physiol. (Lond.)*, *153*, 113
Hewer, A. J. H. and Keele, C. A. (1948). *Lancet, ii*, 683
Hewer, A. J. H., Keele, K. D., Keele, C. A. and Natham, P. W. (1949). *Lancet, i*, 431
Hill, D. (1970). In *Pain in Disablement*. Bradley, W. H. (editor). London: Action for
    the crippled child monograph
Hill, H. E., Kornetsky, C. H., Flanary, H. G. and Wikler, A. (1952). *J. Clin. Invest.*,
    31, 473
Hill, R. C. and Turner, P. (1969). *J. Clin. Pharmacol.*, *9*, 321

Hollander, E. (1939). *J. Lab. Clin. Med.*, *24*, 537

Houde, R. W., Rasmussen, L. H. and La Due, J. S. (1948). *Ann. N.Y. Acad. Sci.*, *51*, 161

Houde, R. W., Wallenstein, S. L. and Rogers, A. (1960). *Clin. Pharmacol. Therap.*, *1*, 163

Huskisson, E. C. (1973). Unpublished observations

Huskisson, E. C. (1974). *Brit. J. Clin. Pharmacol.*, in press

Huskisson, E. C. and Grayson, M. F. (1974). *Brit. J. Clin. Pharmacol.*, In press

Huskisson, E. C. and Hart, F. D. (1971). *Medicine and Hygiene*, *29*, 2054

Huskisson, E. C. and Hart, F. D. (1972). *Brit. med. J.*, *4*, 193

Huskisson, E. C., Shenfield, G. M., Taylor, R. T. and Hart, F. D. (1970). *Rheumatology phys. Med. suppl.*, 88

Huskisson, E. C., Taylor, R. T., Burston, D., Chuter, P. J. and Hart, F. D. (1970). *Ann. rheum. Dis.*, *29*, 393

Huskisson, E. C., Wojtulewski, J. A., Berry, H., Scott, P. J., Hart, F. D. and Balme, H. W. (1974). *Brit. Med. J.*, In press

Iggo, A. (1972). In *Pain*, Janzen, R., Keidel, W. D., Herz, A. and Steichele, C. (editors). London: Churchill Livingstone

Ivy, A. C., Goetzl, F. R., Harris, S. C. and Burrill, D. Y. (1944). *Quart. Bull. Northw. Univ. med. Sch.*, *18*, 298

Kamerman, J. S. (1966). *Ann. rheum. Dis.*, *25*, 361

Kantor, T. G., Sunshine, A., Laska, E., Meisner, M. and Hopper, M. (1966). *Clin. Pharm. Therap.*, *7*, 447

Kast, E. C. (1968). *Med. Clin. N. America*, *52*, 23

Keele, C. A. and Armstrong, D. (1964). *Substances Producing Pain and Itch*. Baltimore: Williams and Wilkins

Keele, K. D. (1948). *Lancet*, **ii**, 6

Keele, K. D. (1954). *Lancet*, **i**, 636

Keele, K. D. (1962). In *The Assessment of Pain in Man and Animals*, Keele, C. A. and Smith, R. (editors). London: Livingstone

Keele, K. D. (1968). *Brit. med. J.*, *1*, 670

Kennard, M. A. (1959). *J. Clin. Invest.*, *31*, 245

Kryger, J. and Aggerbeck, B. (1968). *Ugeskr. Laeg.*, *130*, 1014

Lasagna, L. (1964). *Pharm. Rev.*, *16*, 47

Lee, L. E. (1942). *J. Pharmacol.*, *75*, 161

Lee, R. E. and Pfeiffer, C. C. (1951). *J. Appl. Physiol.*, *4*, 193

Lewis, T., Pickering, G. W. and Rothschild, P. (1931). *Heart*, *15*, 359

Libman, E. (1934). *J. Amer. med. Ass.*, *102*, 335

Lim, R. K. S. and Guzman, F. (1968). In *Pain*, Soulairac, A., Cahn, J. and Charpentier, J. (editors). London and New York: Academic Press

Loan, W. B. and Dundee, J. W. (1967). *Practitioner*, *198*, 759

Marshall, H. R. (1894). *Pain, Pleasure and Aesthetics*. London: Macmillan

Masson, A. H. B. (1962). *Curr. Res. Anaesth.*, *41*, 615

McCarty, C. S. and Drake, R. L. (1956). *Proc. Mayo Clinic*, *31*, 208

Melzack, R. and Wall, P. D. (1965). *Science*, *150*, 971

Merskey, H., Gillis, A. and Marszalek, K. S. (1962). *J. Ment. Sci.*, *108*, 347

Merskey, H. and Spear, F. G. (1964). *Brit. J. Soc. Clin. Psychol.*, *3*, 130

Merskey, H. and Spear, F. G. (1967). *Pain: Psychological and Psychiatric Aspects*. London: Baillière, Tindall and Cassell

Noordenbos, W. (1968). In *Pain*, Soulairac, A., Cahn, J. and Charpentier, J. (editors). London and New York: Academic Press

Notermans, S. L. H. (1967). *Neurology*, *17*, 58

Parkhouse, J. and Holmes, C. M. (1963). *Proc. Roy. Soc. Med.*, *56*, 579

Pelner, L. (1941). *J. Lab. Clin. Med.*, *27*, 248

Schmidt, R. F. (1972). In *Pain*, Janzen, R., Keidel, W. D., Herz, A. and Steichele, C. London: Churchill Livingstone

Scott, J. T. (1965). *Ann. rheum. Dis.*, *14*, 526

Seevers, M. H. and Pfeiffer, C. C. (1936). *J. Pharmacol.*, *56*, 166

Sherman, E. D. (1943). *Canad. Med. Ass. J.*, *48*, 437

Smith, R. (1967). *Proc. Roy. Soc. Med.*, *60*, 415

Smith, G. M. and Beecher, H. K. (1969). *Clin. Pharmacol. Therap.*, *10*, 213

Sternbach, R. A. and Tursky, B. (1965). *Psychophysiology*, *1*, 241

Strong, C. A. (1895). *Psychol. Rev.*, *2*, 329

Suchman, E. (1965). *J. Health and Hum. Behav.*, *6*, 114

Swerdlow, M., Murray, A. and Daw, R. H. (1963). *Acta anaesth. Scand.*, *7*, 1

Szasz, T. S. (1957). *Pain and Pleasure*. London: Tavistock

Traut, E. F. and Passarelli, E. W. (1957). *Ann. rheum. Dis.*, *16*, 18

Trotter, W. (1921). *Med. Sci.*, *4*, 43

Vane, J. R. (1971). *Nature New Biology*, *231*, 232

von Frey, M. (1894). *Bev. d. legl. sachs. Ges. d. Wiss.*, 283

Wall, P. D. and Sweet, W. H. (1967). *Science*, *155*, 108

Wells, H. S. (1947). *Archs. phys. Med.*, *28*, 135

Wilder, R. M. (1940). *Proc. Mayo Clinic*, *15*, 551

Wolff, B. B. (1968). *Arth. Rheum.*, *11*, 519

Wolff, B. B. and Jarvik, M. E. (1964). *Amer. J. Psychol.*, *77*, 589

Wolff, B. B., Kantor, T. G., Jarvik, M. E. and Laska, E. (1969). *Clin. Pharmacol. Therap.*, *10*, 217

Woolfe, G. and Macdonald, A. D. (1944). *J. Pharmacol.*, *80*, 300

Woollard, H. H., Weddell, G. and Harpman, J. A. (1940). *J. Anat.*, *74*, 413

Zborowsky, M. (1952). *Journal of Social Issues*, *8*, 16

2

A Psychiatric Perspective
on Pain and its Control*

Thomas S. Szasz

I

Pain is a universal human experience. This makes it both very easy and very difficult to talk about it. On the one hand, everyone knows something about pain, at least about his own; on the other hand, different persons have often different interests in and attitudes toward pain and hence use the word 'pain' in different ways. For example, to the physician, pain is principally a problem of diseases or injuries that trigger nervous impulses; to the patient, it is principally a problem of discomfort and suffering which warns him of a malfunctioning of his body; and to the theologian, it is principally a problem of guilt and punishment (Szasz, 1957). Actually, each of these persons attends to a different object: the physician, to the patient's body as a biological machine; the patient, to his own body as a personal possession; and the theologian, to the experiences of individuals as moral agents vis-à-vis God. Furthermore, each of these perspectives entails certain kinds of interventions as the appropriate methods for the control of pain.

What is the psychiatric perspective on pain? And the psychiatric attitude on appropriate methods for controlling pain? These questions, and the problem of pain in general which prompts them, confront us with some of the most basic problems in medical and psychiatric epistemology — namely, the problem of pain as a language (Szasz, 1961).

* Portions of this chapter have appeared previously in Szasz, T. S. (1968). The Psychology of Persistent Pain, in Soulairac, A. et al., Eds., Pain, London: Academic Press, pp. 93–113, and are used here by kind permission of the publisher.

II

Although I shall not define pain—because I do not believe that all 'painful' states contain some essence, 'pain', that is definable—I would like to explain my use of the term. In referring to my own pains I shall mean that *I feel pain*; in referring to the pains of others, I shall mean that they report, to me or someone else, that *they feel pain*.

This approach may seem wholly subjective and hence inappropriate for scientific work. I believe, and I hope to show, that it is neither. The anatomist may, to be sure, study brains; the physiologist, electric impulses in nerves; and the pharmacologist, the responses of subjects to drugs. But these men do not, in my opinion, observe or study pain any more than engineers who build television transmitters and repairmen who fix television receivers observe or study the events that newscasters report on the screen (Szasz, 1973). The structure of the human body is an important and interesting subject; and obviously, without bodies we could have neither selves nor pains. It is easy to conclude from this that pains are 'caused' by injuries to the body, or, more specifically, by certain kinds of nervous stimuli. This is the familiar model of pain as the ringing telephone bell, with the caller as the painful stimulus, the wires as peripheral nerves, and the telephone receiver as the brain. This model helps us to understand and control many common medical situations—for example, the pain of a fractured arm; but it fails us utterly in many other kinds of situations—for example, the pain of hypochondriasis.

A dramaturgic-existential approach to pain recognizes not only man's subjectivity, but also his profound dependence on other persons. In other words, existence is at once private and public, concealed and revealed—depending on the identities of actor and audience. Private experiences are those in which we attend to our own inner plays, as in dreams. When we display these experiences by words or action, our selves become actors in a public drama witnessed by and involving others. In short, my approach borrows psychoanalysis from psychiatry, role theory from sociology, and existentialism and linguistic analysis from philosophy. Out of this mixture, I have tried to fashion a coherent dramaturgic-existentialist perspective on personal experience and conduct, including that which we call 'pain'.

III

Foremost among the properties that characterize human beings is consciousness. The question, "How do I know that I am conscious?" has two classical answers, and one modern. Descartes said, "Cogito ergo sum". This may be paraphrased as, "I am aware of my thoughts, therefore I am conscious, therefore I exist". Others, pleading for the supremacy of emotion over thought, have argued that we infer our existence most directly from our consciousness of feelings. These two views of consciousness have been effectively refuted by Gilbert Ryle, who showed that ideas and affects are not objects displayed in the store windows of our minds, where, with the aid of our 'inner eyes' — called introspection — we inspect them. According to Ryle, to be conscious means being conscious of *something*; this means *attending* to or *heeding* something:

> ". . . so far from heeding being a sort of inspecting or monitoring, inspecting and monitoring are themselves special exercises of heed; since whether a person is described literally or metaphorically as a spectator, it is always significant to ask whether he has been a careful or careless spectator, a vigilant or drowsy one" (Ryle, 1949).

One of the things to which human beings pay attention is emotions. Since pain is a complex emotion (I distinguish it from discomfort or distress, which are the proper terms for describing the unpleasant affects of the newborn), a psychological approach to the study of pain must consist largely of observing the ways in which people pay attention to or heed pain in various situations.

An emotion, I wish to emphasize, is not something that happens to a person. It is not — as textbooks of psychophysics or physiology describe a so-called sensation — a specific kind of 'stimulus' impinging on its appropriate central 'receptor organ'. This language is appropriate to telephones, but not to people. This is not the way human pain, especially if it is persistent, is generated and maintained.

"It is man", said Sartre in *Sketch for a theory of emotions*, ". . . who assumes his emotion and emotion is therefore an organized form of human experience". This element of *activity* is specifically stressed for pain by Achelis, who asserts that pain "is not a sensation: . . . [it] is experiencing a performance of the organism". And Sartre observes that there can be no emotion without signification: "Emotion does not exist, considered as a physical phenomenon, for a body cannot be emotional, not being able to attribute meaning to its own manifestations" (*op. cit.*, p. 29). To assert that it is only its particular meaning that renders an experience 'painful' is tautological; and yet it must be said in order to clarify the endlessly repeated phrases in medical, physiological and surgical texts which report about men having 'painful wounds' but no 'pain', or of individuals having undiminished 'pain sensations' but diminished 'reactions to pain' (Beecher, 1959). All such accounts suffer from mixing the vocabularies of physics and psychology. The medical investigator tends to speak in this double language partly from force of habit; and partly from an effort — at once unnecessary and misleading — to relate the subject's report of pain to a malfunctioning of his body. This effort must be relinquished, or at least suspended, if we are to penetrate deeper into the personal meaning and social significance of painful feelings and reports of pain.

IV

The primary social function of the physician is said to be the relief of pain. As a rule, the physician tries, first, to diagnose the patient's illness, partly from pain and partly from other symptoms and signs; and, second, to control the pain by treating the disease which causes it. For example, if a patient with myocardial insufficiency complains of pain in the left arm, the physician does not amputate the painful extremity: instead, he seeks to promote improved coronary circulation; he may also administer drugs to dull the patient's attention to pain. The physician's difficulties in relieving pain in this way do not concern us here. We are interested rather in those situations where pain does not point to an underlying bodily disease and where treatment does not attenuate or relieve pain.

The standard therapeutic methods of medicine fail in two types of situations — not just in practice, but in principle. The first is exemplified by the individual who is physically healthy but nevertheless complains of pain. A man may thus complain of pain in his penis and implore the doctor to 'cut it off'. If his request is not met, he may amputate his own penis. To be sure, such persons are diagnosed as suffering from the 'disease' called 'schizophrenia'. But does schizophrenia 'cause' and 'explain' pain in the penis in the sense in which coronary insufficiency 'causes' and 'explains' pain in the left arm? And can 'schizophrenia' be treated and thus the penile pain be relieved? The answer to both of these questions is: No. In this type of situation, the physician is not confronted with a disease that causes or is manifested by pain; instead, he is confronted simply with *pain*, or with a *complaint of pain*, or with a *painful person*, or, last but not least, with a person who tries to make the physician suffer. The treatment or control of pain here poses a different problem from that encountered in standard medical practice.

The second type of pain situation in which the usual medical approach fails is exemplified by the severely depressed and agitated person who complains of annoying bodily feelings, such as itching, headaches, lack of appetite, insomnia, backache and so forth. Such a person has adopted—fully or partly, permanently or temporarily—the career of being sick and in pain. He does not want his pains allayed or relieved. What is the physician's task in this situation? *Whose* pain should he control: The patient's? That of his relatives, tortured by the patient's complaints? Or his own, generated by his inability to help the patient?

These examples place the problem of the control of pain in its proper perspective. Unless we wish to restrict our attention to purely medical and surgical considerations, we cannot even speak here of the 'treatment' of pain: for 'treatment' implies that the pain resides in a particular person, the patient, and can be influenced by altering the anatomy or chemistry of his body. But what about those patients whose pain is not of this kind? The experiences of these individuals and their relations to others, especially members of their family and doctors, is the proper concern of psychiatrists.

V

One thing strikes the careful observer of patients with chronic pain, especially in cases without organic illness: it is that they are individuals who have made a career of suffering. At one time such persons may have been attorneys or architects, busboys or businessmen, models or maids; but when their careers fail or no longer suffice to sustain them, they become 'painful persons'; or to paraphrase the French diagnostic term *tic douloureux*, they become *hommes douloureux*; or to put it in Latin, they become *homini dolorosi*.

The view that being in pain may be a career was actually described — without putting it quite so bluntly — by Freud himself in *Studies on Hysteria* (Breuer and Freud, 1893–95). This is how Freud summed up his understanding of why Fräulein Elizabeth von R. complained of pains without being demonstrably ill and which yielded to no medical treatment:

> "Here, then, was the unhappy story of this proud girl with her longing for love. Unreconciled to her fate, embittered by the failure of all her little schemes for re-establishing the family's former glories, with those she loved dead or gone away or estranged, unready to take refuge in the love of some unknown man — she had lived for eighteen months in almost complete seclusion, with nothing to occupy her but the care of her mother and her own pains".

This, in my opinion, is one of the finest and most important paragraphs in all of Freud's writings. Free of psychiatric jargon and of psychoanalytic pretense, Freud here reminds us, in plain but persuasive language, that playing the sick role may, for some people some time, be the most gratifying pursuit open to them.·

When referred to psychiatrists, patients of this kind are diagnosed as hysterics, hypochondriacs, schizophrenics, depressives, and so forth. These terms help neither patients nor doctors. The humanistic physician must try to understand such persons and see their life from *their* perspective, not his. To choose pain, suffering and doctoring as a career means attending to the dysfunctions of the body and their repair. Many physicians dislike treating such patients. That is their privilege. A physician is not obligated to treat anyone whom he does not wish to accept as a patient, except in certain emergency situations. He may either refuse to accept the person as his patient or, if he has accepted him, he may dismiss him from his care. To my mind, this is no more of a 'rejection' of the patient than his being told that a mailman does not deliver cars. On the contrary, such a communication is an important clarification of the physician's role. Indeed, I believe that the imperfect definition of the role of healer in contemporary society is an important reason for the prevalence of certain kinds of painful complaints.

This perspective on the problem of pain opens up certain hitherto unrevealed similarities between 'painful persons' and others (both 'normal' and 'pathological') characterized by excessive or too intense attending. The mathematician, for example, attends intently to unsolved problems of algebra; the musician, to his yet-to-be-composed symphony; the engineer, to plans for his new bridge; the detective, to his elusive criminal; the politician, to his 'communist' or 'fascist enemies'; the phobic, to his fears; the Don Juan, to his sexual appetite and its satisfaction; the paranoid, to his persecutors; and so forth.

When pain is chronic and 'unbearable', so that it pre-empts the patient's complete attention, the situation resembles certain severe 'mental illnesses', especially 'compulsive' states, 'agitated depressions', and 'schizophrenic delusions'. In each of these situations, we are confronted by individuals who, in the older language of psychiatry, are 'monomaniacal': that is to say, they have only one interest in life. Such persons are interested in nothing but their pet subject; and they impose it on anyone who happens to come into their orbit. This is what makes them social nuisances. However, by looking at this kind of behavior with some detachment, we can see how it resembles the behavior of many other persons — especially that of the political leader or religious zealot. Each of these persons is passionately convinced of the correctness of his own point of view and its overriding importance in world affairs; and each tries to impose it on as many other persons as he can. Those who possess political or religious power have the means to do so: they can command attentive audiences and compliant followers. Those who lack such power often have no one who will listen to them; hence, they resort to interpersonal coercion. This is exemplified by the conduct of many people said to be 'mentally ill'. The 'paranoid schizophrenic', for example, may believe that his penis is the devil's hiding-place and try to convince the physician that it should therefore be amputated.

'The persuader', as Minogue (1963) correctly emphasizes, "is not a man who must find solutions for problems, but one who must construct problems to fit pre-existing solutions".

As pain constitutes the career of *l'homme douloureux*, so its diagnosis and relief constitute the career of many physicians. The passion of patients trying to persuade physicians to engage in this or that pain-relieving intervention is matched only by the passion of physicians recommending this or that pain-allaying treatment. Just as the seriousness of the patient's devotion to suffering is measured by his resistance to relinquishing his chosen career, so the seriousness of the physician's devotion to relieving pain is measured by his resistance to admitting defeat in his struggle against pain. Only in this light can we understand the wide variation among physicians in their attitude toward the patient with 'untreatable' chronic pain. Some — especially neurosurgeons — never give up; they command numerous pain-relieving strategies from operations on peripheral nerves to lobotomy. Others — especially general practitioners and internists — try to alleviate the patient's suffering, but only up to a point; when their drugs and patience are exhausted, they give up. Still others — especially psychoanalysts — do not even try, in a sense, to relieve the patient's pain; they will listen and talk to the patient, but not do anything to increase or diminish his pain; their effort is confined to helping the patient help himself — if that is what he wants — to exchange his career of suffering for another occupation.

The choice of each of these careers — both as patient and doctor — is a personal matter. Severe, chronic illness does not necessarily lead to a career of pain, if the individual has something better to do with his life than to suffer. During his last years, Freud was afflicted with cancer of the oral cavity; he attended to his work, however, not to his illness. When he was younger, and the significance of his work was less secure, he was hypochondriacal. On the other hand, people free of physical disease often suffer from the most intractable types of pain. In such cases, unless the patient can find something more interesting and worthwhile to attend to, the career of pain is apt to last till death.

The physician's choice of the type of pain-relieving he will engage in is also a personal matter. I doubt that doctors become psychoanalysts, internists, or neurosurgeons because they come to believe that the methods of one of these specialties is more effective than that of another for relieving human suffering. It is rather the young physician's attitude toward suffering — and his efforts to master it by reflective acceptance, understanding, and distraction, or by more active methods of persuasion, drugs, and surgery — that determine his occupational choice and his subsequent conduct in the medical situation. For it is not only that "it is the sick man who creates the doctor" (Sartre, *op. cit*, pp. 103–104), but also that the doctor creates the sick man. The "social and material relation" [between doctor and patient], observes Sartre, "is affirmed in practice as a bond even more intimate than the sexual act; but this intimacy is realized only by activities, and precise, original techniques engaging both persons. . . . Doctor and patient form a couple united by a common enterprise". It is for this reason that the humanistic understanding and mastery of pain requires attention to the role and conduct of the physician no less than to the experiences and diseases of the patient.

VI

From the point of view of the experiencing person, there is no such thing as 'psychogenic pain'. Individuals always ascribe their pains to some disease or dysfunction of their bodies. Hence, the terms 'organic' and 'psychogenic' must be recognized as adjectives of a particular kind, resembling terms like 'normal' and 'psychotic', 'enlightened' and 'reactionary'. In each of these pairs, the first member expresses approval, and the second disapproval, of the experience or conduct which it modifies; this valuation, moreover, is so conceived and is so intense that in ordinary usage a person would never describe his pain as 'psychogenic', his conduct as 'psychotic', or his political views as 'reactionary'; these terms may be used, however, by one person to describe, and usually to condemn, the experience, conduct or politics of another.

It is clear, then, that 'psychogenic pain' and 'organic pain' are not two kinds of pains in the sense in which English and French are two kinds of languages. Instead, they resemble the expressions 'beautiful painting' and 'ugly painting'; these are judgments which an observer might render about different canvases, or which different observers might render about the same canvas.

Rarely is language used to frame a pure description. Often its purpose is to exert some kind of influence. This is especially true of the language for describing and classifying pain. Simply put, the patient in pain wants to know what ails him; and the physician wants to know what part of the patient's body is injured or diseased. In this situation, the pain is like a *corpus delicti*, and the physician like a detective in search of a culprit, that is, a pain-producing lesion.

From a dramaturgic perspective, the problem of distinguishing between organic or real pain and psychogenic or imaginary pain appears in a quite different light. Instead of distinguishing between two types of pains, we distinguish between two types of bodies: those that are injured or diseased, and those that are alleged or seem to be but are not. As Gilbert Ryle (1949) points out,

> "There are not two species of murderers, those who murder people, and those who act the parts of murderers on the stage; for these last are not murderers at all. They do not commit murders which have the elusive attribute of being shams; they pretend to commit ordinary murders, and pretending to murder entails, not murdering, but seeming to murder. As mock-murders and not murders, so imagined sights and sounds are not sights and sounds. . . . There is no answer to the spurious question, 'Where have you deposited the victim of your mock-murder?' since there was no victim. There is no answer to the question, 'Where do the objects reside that we fancy we see?' since there are no such objects".

The physician-detective's problem is similar and yields to the same analysis. There are not two species of sick people, those who suffer from pains due to bodily lesions, and those who suffer from pains due to mental lesions; for these last are not patients at all. Pains that are imagined, hallucinated or pretended — call them what we may — are not the signs of bodily diseases, just as actors pretending to be corpses are not the signs of ordinary crimes. As mock-murders have no victims, so mock-pains have no lesions.

This view of so-called psychogenic pain resembles, of

course, certain older concepts of malingering, conversion hysteria, and hypochondriasis, according to which patients of this sort are like impostors: though healthy, they deceive the physician (or even themselves) with faked illness. This view is substantially correct, but incomplete. It neglects the complementary deception of patients by physicians, which is the soil in which the patient's deception grows and flowers.

Physicians have always tried to heal men both in body and soul. Until modern times, the medical man could actually do little in the way of organic treatment; the benefit he brought to his patients was largely personal. The modern physician, on the other hand, though skilled in a variety of highly specific medical techniques, continues to insist that his professional competence is not limited to the cure of bodies but encompasses the cure of souls as well. This definition of the doctor's role is a deception no less grave than that of the malingerer or hysteric. The malingerer says "I am sick", when, in fact, he is not; the (non-psychiatric) physician says "I am an expert in the diagnosis and treatment not only of bodily diseases but of personal problems as well", when, in fact, he is not; and the psychiatrist says "I am an expert in the diagnosis and treatment not only of mental diseases but of bodily ailments as well", when, in fact, he is not. The malingerer plays the sick role; the (non-psychiatric) physician, the role of the psychotherapist; and the psychiatrist, that of the physician. The upshot is a vast confusion of roles, each impostor trying desperately, often coercively, to authenticate his role and compel its acceptance by his audience.

It is all as if detectives and drama critics on the one hand, and gangsters and actors on the other, were to confuse and exchange their roles. Detectives would then try to solve mock-murders; drama critics would pursue real murderers; gangsters would perform on the stage as actors; and actors would commit real crimes offstage. This kind of confusion and deception flourishes in contemporary medical practice, where the same individuals try to combine the roles of physician and priest, and purport to be able to cure both bodies and souls. Indeed, some proponents of 'holistic' or 'psychosomatic' medicine regard the abolition of all distinction between suffering due to bodily disease and to life experiences as the most important task facing their movement. They have succeeded to a remark-able extent in convincing the public, and themselves, that the physician is, or ought to be, an omni-competent healer whose therapeutic interest is attracted equally by bodily pains and personal suffering.

VII

My comments about mutual deception between patients and doctors in situations of so-called 'psychogenic' pain may be corroborated by patients, through introspection; by physicians, through candid observation and self-observation; and by the general reader, through perusal of medical, surgical and psychiatric writings on pain. I shall quote from and comment on some passages from an article which, in contrast to the specifically medical, surgical or psychological, exemplifies the so-called psychosomatic approach to this problem.

Tinling and Klein (1966) report their experiences with 'fourteen men with intractable psychogenic pain'. The setting in which their observations were made was that of a 'Medical–Psychiatric Liaison Service' in a large, university-affiliated medical center, in which the authors held appointments in both the Medical and Psychiatric Departments. The descrip-tion of their patients is unremarkable. Of special interest to us are their recommendations for treatment.

"Treatment is very difficult", they write. "By the time we saw the men, they had usually seen many doctors with little satisfaction. Such individuals seem to have difficulty entering into the doctor–patient relationship, and they seem to provoke rejection on the part of the physician".

What can we infer from these observations? First, that these patients do not make themselves clearly understood by their physicians; and second, that the physicians do not clearly inform the patients that they cannot help them. To assert that such patients have 'difficulty in entering into the doctor–patient relationship', is false. Actually, they enter into the sick-role and into the medical relationship with great ease. The difficulty stems from the fact that their demands are usually frustrated by the physician. For example, the patient may want an operation; the physician, being unable to find bodily lesions to justify it, will refuse to recommend or perform an operation. He will usually do so, because as a physician he feels that he, not the patient, is the proper judge of the kind of treatment necessary. The patient, however, refuses to treat the physician as a medical authority. In short, both patient and physician insist on having their own way; each tries to persuade the other of the validity of his ideas about what is 'wrong', and of the legitimacy of his authority to decide on how to 'correct' it; each refuses to be convinced by the other. The upshot is mutual frustration and antagonism.

Tinling and Klein sense this covert antagonism and struggle for dominance. To resolve it, they recommend that the physician pretend to agree with the patient: "The single most important aspect of treatment is the attitude of the physician. He must believe with the patient that the pain is real. Any indication that the pain is 'imaginary' only humiliates the patient, in a way making him appear to be a liar, and treatment may then be impossible. . . . It also seems wise to avoid hasty referrals, especially to psychiatrists, for these will be seen as rejections, and the patients are not likely to want psychiatric help. (A typical patient's response is to say, 'How can it all be in my head when I hurt here?')".

What do the authors mean when they assert that the physician "must believe . . . that the pain is real?" Evidently they do not mean that he must believe that the patient has 'real' psychogenic pain, although, judging by the title of their article, this is what they, the authors, believe; nor do they propose that this is what the physician tells the patient. They can only mean, then, that the physician should pretend to agree with the patient's interpretation of the nature of the pain; he should play the role of a doctor who accepts the patient's claim to the sick role, authenticated by 'real' bodily illness.

The patient's tactic, and the physician's counter-tactic, as illustrated in the passage cited, exemplify what I call the mutual deception of patients and doctors. The patient deceives the doctor by asserting that his body is sick, when, in fact, his life is askew. The physician deceives the patient by letting him believe that he will treat him for a bodily illness when, in fact, he plans to treat him for mental illness. The patient's strategy is facilitated by framing his complaint in the idiom of body language; the physician's, by assuming the role of doctor.

Patient and physician play complementary roles in this situation. The patient insists that his problem is physical, not mental; the physician insists that he is a medical doctor (neurologist, internist, etc.), not a psychological healer (psychotherapist). Just as pain authenticates that the patient's illness is physical (in a way that anxiety, for example, is not), so it also authenticates the healer's role as medical (in a way that a marital problem, for example, does not). Patient and physician thus engage in a kind of tacit collusion to accept pain, and pain alone, as proof of the 'reality' of bodily illness, and hence as sufficient ground for the patient's adoption of the sick role. The authors thus abandon the traditional medical position according to which the ultimate criterion of bodily illness is not a 'symptom' or complaint (such as pain), but a 'sign' or finding (such as a wound). This is another manifestation of the modern psychiatric tendency to expand the category of illness to include all manner of non-medical problems.

As if realizing, as they must, that their patients are not truly sick, Tinling and Klein recommend that the physician insist that the patient must be physically ill by arguing that there can be no pain without bodily illness. "It seems helpful to point out to the patient", they write, "that some people have pain just as some people have arthritis or rheumatism, and that just as arthritis will wax and wane, so will the pain. If a patient can understand that a doctor does not cure pain, he may be able to see his illness in a better perspective. The patient can be told that the doctor will be his doctor throughout the illness, and that the patient can have some good days and some bad days".

The result of this approach, however, is not that the patient is persuaded to understand that the 'doctor does not cure pain', but rather that the doctor accepts the pain and the patient's view of it without apparent skepticism. This tactic is more helpful for the physician than for the patient: it bolsters the patient's role as a sick person (which may or may not be an advantage for him), while supporting the psychiatrist's role as a doctor (which is likely to be an advantage for him). Nor is this a novel gambit: it is the classic strategy of the alienist who 'accepts' the patient's assertion that he is Napoleon, and, in so doing, codifies the patient's role as 'mad' and his own as 'sane'.

Yet, only by explicitly rejecting the patient's interpretation of his own bodily state does the physician treat him as a responsible person; and only in this way does the physician give the patient an opportunity to match his judgment against that of the physician and to make an informed choice between the two (Szasz, 1965).

VIII

The concept of the painful person' which I am proposing merits a more detailed description and analysis. I can do no more here than to indicate and illustrate the most important features of this phenomenon.

In the history of Western thought, it has been the custom to characterize the specifically 'human' quality of man by his dominant and governing interest. For example, the free citizen of ancient Athens is regarded as the paradigm of political man or *homo politicus*. In this concept, participation in the affairs of the community distinguishes man from the slave, the barbarian, and the animal.

For religious man or *homo theologicus* of medieval Europe, on the other hand, it is the individual's relations to God and Church that determine his status as a human being and impart dignity and significance to him. In this concept, religious faith in Christianity distinguishes man from the unbaptized, the Jew, the heathen, and the animal.

For economic man or *homo economicus* of the eighteenth and nineteenth centuries, finally, it is the individual's relations to goods and services that determine his status as a person. In this concept, the appreciation of and the ability to use capital and labor, work and leisure, characterize man as a 'rational' creature and distinguish him from children, savages, and the insane.

My concept of the 'painful person' — or *homo dolorosus*, or *l'homme douloureux* — is intended as a similar short-hand characterization. It refers to a man whose humanity is intimately related to, or is wholly dependent upon, his being in pain and suffering. In this concept, pain and suffering — rather than political liberty, economic rationalism, or psychological reflectiveness — make man specifically human, and distinguish and raise him above those who — like animals, unconscious persons, or madmen — do not or cannot suffer. To be sure, suffering here connotes not merely 'physical pain' but a condition pervading the subject's entire personality.

This image of man as sufferer has a long history, perhaps as long as recorded history itself. For the Western world, Christianity gave it a powerful impetus and placed upon it a distinctive stamp. Jesus's signal achievement is his boundless suffering: through His suffering, He rescued mankind from sin and became the Savior. The Virgin Mary is called *Mater Dolorosa*: she is the suffering, sorrowful, or painful mother. The classic, Catholic significance of pain and suffering received fresh impetus and meaning from modern rationalism and liberalism. And finally, in our day, it was carried to its absurd, medical–technological limit, through the application of pharmacological and surgical methods to *pain*, rather than to the *person* in pain. As *homo theologicus* required a social milieu pervaded by religious values and dominated by the priest, so *homo dolorosus* requires a social milieu pervaded by medical values and dominated by the physician. Indeed, it is here, and here alone, that this kind of human being can exist and flourish.

We might say — at the risk of caricaturizing the situation — that there is nothing a real physician loves more than a patient who suffers from bodily disease and who complains of pains that point directly to its cause and nature. A patient with 'real' or 'organic' pain is like the true penitent of medieval Christianity: he plays the role of patient 'faithfully', thus allowing the physician to play his role as diagnostician and therapist. Conversely, there is nothing a real physician hates more than a patient who complains falsely of bodily illness (like the 'malingerer') or who, though declared to be ill, refuses to play the sick role (like the 'paranoid schizophrenic'): such individuals are 'medical heretics' who, by refusing to play the role of patient, frustrate the physician in his efforts to play the role of diagnostician and therapist.

The character of contemporary medical mores — which is the social context in which *homo dolorosus* arises and flourishes — is manifested in many ways. Perhaps nothing typifies it more, however, than the physician's disappointment, disapproval and dismay when a person he considers sick neither complains of pain nor regards himself as bodily or mentally ill. The proto-type of this kind of 'patient' today is the 'delinquent' youth. Here is what a college psychiatrist and a college psychologist say about these young people: "Because our contact with these unruly students is so brief, it is difficult for us to gain a complete picture of their personality structure or to come to any real understanding of why they behave the way they do. . . ." This limitation does not prevent them, however, from reaching the confident conclusion that these students "can be diagnosed as suffering from a basic character disorder" (Blaine and McArthur, 1961). Actually, these students do not themselves suffer from anything; they make others, especially college administrators and psychiatrists, suffer.

Just as the medieval witch could commit no graver sin than to be a heretic and yet feel no guilt, so the young trouble-maker in a contemporary medical–psychiatric setting can suffer from no more serious disease than 'mental illness' and yet not complain of suffering! "These students", write Blaine and McArthur, "seldom come to the clinic of their own choice, not because they feel they should go it alone, as the drop-out students so often do, but rather because they do not believe that their difficulties are the result of emotional conflicts. . . . Characteristically, these students prove reluctant to engage in a therapeutic relationship. They do not want to come to the clinic and they tend to deny their difficulties. . . ." It is clear that whatever the students may or may not want in the way of human relationships, the experts are *very eager* to treat them as *patients*, and to *affirm their identity as sick individuals*. I cite this example merely to illustrate the therapeutic pull which physicians exert on society, encouraging persons to experience and present themselves as ill patients: preferably, citizens should complain of pain and should suffer from bodily illness; but, if that is impossible, at least they should complain of 'imaginary pain' and should suffer from 'mental illness'. Only by seeing the 'painful person' against this background of medical expectation can we begin to understand him and his probable fate; and only in this way can we understand the deep-seated resistance, both medical and popular, to accepting pain and suffering as not only the symptom of a disorder, whether bodily or mental — but also as an existential condition, meaningful and significant in its own right; and only thus can we appreciate the ironic consequences of salvationism in politics and therapeutism in medicine which deny the individual, both as citizen and as patient, his inalienable *right to suffer*. No longer will man be allowed to suffer the wounds inflicted on him by the capricious 'slings and arrows of outrageous fortune'; if suffer he must, he will be compelled to undergo the standardized 'treatments' planned for and imposed on him, in the name of freedom and health, by the Therapeutic State.

Psychiatrists often assert that many mental patients 'deny' their illness. What they actually mean and ought to say is that these are individuals who strongly resist being cast into the sick role: Although declared ill by physicians, they do not regard themselves as patients and are especially stubborn about refusing to accept as their doctors the psychiatrists who label them sick. This pan-medical ideology, seeking a limitless expansion of the category of illness, is the basis for our contemporary 'psychosomatic' misinterpretation of pain—that is, the medical and psychiatric presumption that everyone who complains of pain is 'sick'—either bodily or mentally.

By treating all persons who complain of pain and suffering as if they were sick, physicians in effect deny that exaggerated attention to the body and to painful 'sensations' emanating from it may impart meaning and significance to a person's life; hence, it need not constitute illness, or even the symptoms of illness. The medical proclivity for viewing everyone who complains of his body as sick is one aspect of a double denial: physicians deny that suffering may be a meaningful career; at the same time, they maintain that persons to whom they ascribe suffering and sickness but who refuse to play the sick role deny the reality of their diseases. These phenomena signify a covert struggle for power—specifically, for the control of the medical relationship.

IX

Let us now consider the case history of a so-called 'painful person' as presented by two non-psychiatric physicians:

A woman of hysterical temperament began at the age of 16 to complain of abdominal pain so persistently that she accumulated a series of 12–18 abdominal operations, with what might be termed progressive evisceration. Following a trivial head injury, she complained so bitterly of pain in the head that a subtemporal decompression was performed. From 1934 to 1936 she was confined to bed because of agonizing pain in the back and limbs. . . . When we saw her for the first time, she appeared uneasy, would not give her history, and began wincing and overbreathing before the bed covers were turned down. She lay constantly on her left side and cried out if any attempt was made to turn her on her back. She defended herself with her right hand from any examination on her back and when the right hand was restrained and the region of the sacrum was gently stroked, she screamed and trembled violently. On account of exaggeration of the complaints with very little anatomic substrate, a diagnosis of conversion hysteria with polysurgical addiction was made. [The patient was subsequently lobotomized.] (Freeman and Watts, 1950.)

Freeman and Watts regard this woman as having an 'imaginary' illness. The question is: Why do these physicians, and so many others, interpret 'imaginary' illness as itself an illness?

When a man 'imagines' that his girl-friend is the most wonderful person in the world and marries her, we call it 'love'; when a man 'imagines' that the president of his country is a great leader and goes happily off to war because he asks him to, we call it 'patriotism'; but when a man 'imagines' that his body is diseased and complains of pains, we conclude that either *his body is sick* or his *imagination is sick*. In short, as physicians, we do not let *others* imagine that they are ill; and we do not let *ourselves* imagine that some people can imagine (and desire) being sick.

Freeman and Watts are quite explicit about this. "We may say that an individual is suffering from imaginary ills", they write, referring to persons with functional psychoses and psychogenic pains. "Indeed, many people — doctors and laymen alike, and especially friends of the patient — say so either behind his back or actually to his face. . . . If instead of imaginary illnesses we speak of diseased imagination, we are probably no better off in the eyes of the patient, since to him his experiences are intensely real. . . . Nevertheless, the question of imagination in the onset and development of these mental ills cannot be taken too lightly. Indeed, in some instances it seems to be the outstanding feature whether or not the patient will admit it. It is in the instances in which insight into the condition is more or less lost that the clearest examples of a diseased imagination — or, if we will speak of it so, an imaginary illness — are presented to the physician".

Is there a difference between an 'imaginary illness' and a 'diseased imagination'? Yes, indeed. An 'imaginary' object differs from its 'real' counterpart mainly in the response each calls forth from the audience before whom it is displayed. A stage-murder evokes applause or boos for the actor, not cries for his arrest. Curiously, physicians never recommend treating mock-illnesses in this way. If an illness is imaginary—as Freeman and Watts at first suggest—then it follows that the last thing the physician should do is to treat the subject as a patient! Doing so renders the sickness real, and its bearer a genuine patient; it is like accepting a well executed forgery of a Rembrandt as a masterpiece and hailing its painter as a great artist. To be sure, it is not wholly irrational to act this way. But it is confusing, especially when it is followed by fresh attempts to declare the illness not quite real but 'mental', and its bearer not really a patient but 'insane'. This would correspond to accepting faked Rembrandts as masterpieces, and then having separate rooms in a museum — some for real Rembrandts, and others for forged ones. This, of course, is exactly what we do in contemporary hospitals: we have two sets of wards, some for patients with real diseases, and others for those with faked ones.

There is another way for physicians to respond to individuals who, in their judgment, suffer from imaginary illnesses or display faked diseases. Instead of treating such individuals as sick, physicians could inform them that they consider them well (or, at least not sick). This would leave physicians free to treat only those patients whom they consider really ill; and it would leave persons with imaginary illnesses free to proceed as they wish. One of the reasons physicians do not conduct themselves in this way is because it would be contrary to their economic self-interest. Instead, they treat pretended illness as the sign of an illness or as an illness itself. The semantic and strategic value of Freeman and Watts's concept of a 'diseased imagination' now becomes clear. Since the objects physicians treat are diseased bodies, it requires only an expansion of the category of objects that may be 'diseased' (from bodies to minds and imaginations) to render the bearers of such diseases sick, and hence fit subjects for medical treatment. The concepts of 'mental illness', 'psychogenic pain' and 'diseased imagination' fulfill this function admirably. They enable us to define persons whose main interests are their bodies and their pains as also sick and in need of medical care. Indeed, these concepts suffice to justify all manner of psychiatric interventions—from commitment, to drugs, to lobotomy, with or without consent of the 'patient'. If, say Freeman and Watts, a person imagines that some part of his body is diseased, when in fact it is not, it would be foolish to operate on these parts. The diseased imagination is in the head. But, "If the trouble is in the head, why work on the belly?"

X

Our views on the control of pain rest, and are largely determined by, our views on the nature of pain. I have briefly noted what I regard as the distinctively psychiatric perspective on pain, emphasizing particularly the experiential meaning and significance of pain for the patient. The essential difference between the approaches to pain appropriate in medicine and surgery on the one hand, and in psychiatry on the other, lies, in my opinion, in that, whereas in the former fields we may properly speak of the 'control of pain', in the latter we must speak instead of the control or self-control of 'persons who complain of pain'. Among such persons, I have called special attention to those with chronic pain but without demonstrable bodily illness, whose suffering may constitute their career. When faced with such a 'painful person', the psychiatrist must choose among several courses open to him: he may refuse to accept him as a patient; he may accept him and undertake to 'treat' him despite the patient's apparent desire to retain his painful identity; or he may accept him for 'treatment' but insist that the patient choose whether he wishes to remain as he is or change.

The first situation requires no further comment. The second often results in a progressively anatagonistic relationship between patient and psychiatrist, the former escalating his painful complaints as the latter escalates his 'therapeutic' assaults on them; such encounters, like bad marriages, often end in divorce, the patient being 'referred' to a neurosurgeon. The third situation is simply an application of a certain kind of psychoanalytic posture to patients whose predominant problems are pain. The psychoanalyst tries to avoid the impasses that characterize the relationship between patients of this sort and their physicians: he does so by treating the client as a person responsible for his life rather than as a patient not responsible for his lesion; by treating pain as an idiom rather than an illness; and by substituting his own dialectic and discursive language for the client's rhetoric and nondiscursive language (Szasz, 1968). If such an enterprise is successful, it is not because the therapist has succeeded in controlling the patient's pain, but because the patient has decided to become another kind of person.

REFERENCES

Achelis, quoted in Buytendijk, J. J. (1943). *Pain: Its Modes and Functions*, trans. by E. O'Shiel, Chicago: University of Chicago Press, 1962, p. 115

Beecher, H. K. (1959). *Measurement of Subjective Responses*. New York: Oxford University Press

Blaine, G. B. Jr. and McArthur, C. C. (editors) (1961). *Emotional Problems of the Student*. New York: Appleton-Century-Crofts, p. 100

Breuer, J. and Freud, S. (1893–95). *Studies on Hysteria*, in *The Standard Edition of the Complete Psychological Works of Sigmund Freud*, London: Hogarth Press, 1955, Vol. II, pp. 143–144

Freeman, W. and Watts, J. W. (1950). *Psychosurgery in the Treatment of Mental Disorders and Intractable Pain*, 2nd Edition. Springfield, Ill.: Thomas, pp. 354–355

Minogue, K. R. (1963). *The Liberal Mind*. London: Methuen, p. 129

Ryle, G. (1949). *The Concept of Mind*. London: Hutchinson's University Library, p. 137

Sartre, J.-P. (1939). *Sketch for a Theory of the Emotions*, trans. by P. Mairet. London: Methuen, p. 28

Szasz, T. S. (1957). *Pain and Pleasure*. New York: Basic Books; London: Tavistock

Szasz, T. S. (1961). *The Myth of Mental Illness*. New York: Hoeber-Harper; London: Paladin (1972); Second Revised Edition, New York: Harper & Row (1974)

Szasz, T. S. (1965). *The Ethics of Psychoanalysis*. New York: Basic Books; London: Routledge & Kegan Paul, 1974

Szasz, T. S. (1968). Hysteria, in *Internat. Encycl. of the Social Sciences*. New York: Macmillan & Free Press, Vol. 7, pp. 47–52

Szasz, T. S. (1973). Mental illness as a metaphor, *Nature* (Lond.), *242*, 305

Tinling, D. C. and Klein, R. F. (1966). Psychogenic pain and aggression, *Psychosom. Med.*, *28*, 738

3

The Control of Pain
in the Rheumatic Disorders

F. Dudley Hart

The rheumatic diseases cover a very large part of the field of
medicine (Hart, 1971), inflammatory, degenerative, traumatic
and infective conditions comprising around 160 or more
different entities (Huskisson and Hart, 1973). Some are acute
and self-terminating, for instance rubellar arthropathy and
acute gout: some abate gradually over a period of a few or
several weeks, for example the arthropathy of sarcoidosis and
many cases of Brodie's (Reiter's) disease. Many, however,
persist as chronic disorders for many months, many years or
the rest of the patient's lifetime, seeming to continue in varying
degrees of activity and subactivity, partial remission being
followed by relapse and a return of symptoms. It is this hard
core of chronic remitting-relapsing rheumatic disease which
causes the most persistent pain and suffering. The rheumatic
disorders cause more time off work and more disability than
any other group of diseases, with the possible exception of
psychiatric disorders, and no other group of patients have more
persistent discomfort as a day to day part of their regular
existence. As one patient said "I open my eyes in the morning
and say 'O God, not another day' and in the evening when I
return to bed 'Dear God, not another night' ". It is this
relentless and remorseless persistence of unremitting pain
which saps what optimism and resilience is left in these gallant
sufferers. These patients live with pain, with the anxiety and
depression that goes with it, with disability and with much
frustration, with, in a word, suffering. Many refuse regular
analgesics as they prefer to have the pain unmodified and un-
mixed with sickness, nausea, headaches, bowel disturbance,
singing in the ears and various other overtones of their daily
drug therapy.

The commonest long-lasting painful rheumatic conditions are:

(1) rheumatoid arthritis;

(2) other sero-negative inflammatory arthropathies;

(3) osteoarthrosis, particularly of hip and knee; and

(4) backaches due to degenerative spinal lesions of different kinds.

As these four groups constitute the main therapeutic problem, they will be considered first.

Rheumatoid arthritis

The patient with rheumatoid arthritis may suffer from the condition for only a few days, weeks or months, but all too often it persists in different grades of activity for many years and often for life. It is, in lay terms, a long pain. It is a cocktail of a number of different ingredients:

(1) local pain in joints and surrounding tissues due to swelling and stretching of inflamed tissues;

(2) local pain on movement due to chronic changes in, and disorganization of, articular tissues;

(3) systemic illness, with fever, tachycardia, anorexia, loss of weight, anemia and sometimes mal-or under-nutrition;

(4) anxiety and depression;

(5) in severe cases extra-articular rheumatoid changes causing pains of different quality, e.g. pericarditis, pleurisy, ischemic changes in extremities, Sjögren's and Felty's syndromes; and finally

(6) therapeutic overtones of dyspepsia (salicylates and other anti-inflammatory agents), constipation (codeine), diarrhea (the anthranilates, mefenamic and flufenamic acids), Cushing's disease (corticosteroids, corticotrophin and tetracosactrin), necrotizing papillitis (compound analgesic tablets), headaches and various unpleasant cerebral sensations (indomethacin), blurred and impaired vision (chloroquin) and other more vague and less easily described symptoms of drug intolerance.

As there is no such thing as an untreated rheumatoid arthritic patient, there are few who never suffer any of this last group of symptoms arising from at least three of the above six groups. The discomfort suffered is therefore a complex one, often difficult to explain to the patient's physician who is, regrettably, often unanxious to hear more complaints from one already very truly and genuinely polysymptomatic. As our first patients said of their recently developed peripheral rheumatoid neuropathy "It's a new feeling, doctor, and it's different; it's not the usual arthritic pain". One other factor to be considered in this disorder is the pain threshold (Huskisson and Hart, 1972a) which has been found to be lowest in those patients confined to house and home and with little to occupy their minds, a group the opposite of the *Typus robustus* of de Haas *et al.* (1973) where the patients, usually male, often self-employed individuals depending on their own initiative and drive, manage to continue to make their active and effective way through life in spite of advanced nodular disease. Huskisson and Hart (1972) found a statistically highly significant relationship between pain threshold and both pain severity and pain duration in patients with rheumatoid arthritis. They also found a statistically significant inverse correlation between pain threshold and total analgesic tablets taken daily. Both articular index, which depends on pain response to pressure applied directly over the joints, and grip strength correlated significantly with pain threshold. These findings in rheumatoid arthritis were entirely different from those in ankylosing spondylitis, as will be discussed later. Although I have personally seen several patients with rheumatoid arthritis where exacerbation of symptoms occurred without measurable increase in signs of disease activity, the increase in symptoms following episodes of distress and domestic upsets, Huskisson and Hart, in the study mentioned above, were not able to identify relapse of rheumatoid disease owing to fall in pain threshold. There is to date little to show that a rheumatoid arthritic with a high pain threshold is any the worse off than one with low pain threshold; what evidence there is points the other way. The practical therapeutic point emerging from this is that it would seem legitimate to attempt to raise pain threshold as part of the therapeutic programme where and if this is possible. This would presumably include encouragement of the patient to lead a life of maximum fulfilment within a certain therapeutic framework, a positive rather than a negative programme of controlled activities.

Let us now take an individual rheumatoid patient and, as it were, dissect him in terms of pain and prescribe accordingly.

1. LOCAL ARTICULAR AND PERIARTICULAR PAIN DUE TO INFLAMMATORY SWELLING

Much of the discomfort in rheumatoid arthritis arises from tissue swelling. The joint capsule is richly endowed with nerve endings as are the tendons at their insertions. The worst time for pain and maximal stiffness and disability for most rheumatoid sufferers is the early morning, when swelling is maximal. The loosening-up or limbering-up time, that is, the time taken in the early morning to recover from the aggravation of pain and stiffness caused by the night's rest, is a useful rough measure of the amount of inflammatory swelling in a given patient. This 'gelling' of the tissues with immobility in sleep is characteristic of all the inflammatory arthropathies. Any effective anti-inflammatory agent must therefore work throughout the 24 hours, and special consideration must be given to the night hours. The patient under effective therapeutic cover can move in sleep without waking up from pain. Anti-inflammatory peripherally acting agents are much more effective than centrally acting analgesics in this respect and heavy sedation aggravates the condition, making the patient more painful and stiff in the early mornings. We feel the most useful agents in diminishing morning stiffness are prednisolone in small dosage, e.g. 5 mg on retiring or the equivalent dose of some other corticosteroid, or 75–100 mg indomethacin in suppository form or by mouth taken with food on retiring. Although blood levels of the drug are minimal by early morning, tissue levels are presumably higher as most patients with active inflammatory disease do derive benefit. Less effective are salicylates, the anthranilates and analgesics such as paracetamol, codeine, dihydrocodeine and dextropropoxyphene, and though longer-acting forms such as aloxiprin and sustained action dextropropoxyphene may be effective in some cases, in many they are not effective enough to control early morning symptoms. The pyrazoles, phenylbutazone and oxyphenbutazone, exert a prolonged even action in rheumatoid arthritis over the 24 hours, but do not usually give the extra booster effect required in the small hours of the early morning.

In the day the first choice is usually aspirin in some form in maximally tolerated dosage, for at 5 g or more in the 24 hours acetylsalicylic acid is an effective anti-inflammatory agent. Unfortunately many patients can only tolerate half this dosage or less and at this lower dosage, although analgesic effects are obtained, demonstrable diminution in joint swelling and stiffness is usually not forthcoming. Corticosteroids, corticotrophin and tetracosactrin, although highly effective anti-inflammatory agents, invariably produce Cushingoid effects if continued in dosage above the equivalent of 7 mg of prednisolone daily.

There is another group of anti-inflammatory agents which act in ways unknown and exert their effects only after several weeks of continued therapy. These are the gold salts, the antimalarials, chloroquin and hydroxychloroquin, and — though still in the stage of experiment rather than orthodox therapy — the immunosuppressive agents and penicillamine. As with all effective agents these have undesirable side-effects, which restrict their usage and limit their application, but all can be considered delayed action long-acting anti-inflammatory agents in rheumatoid arthritis. Anti-inflammatory agents as such are called for where acute inflammatory features are prominent; where rheumatoid disease is largely burnt-out with minimal evidence of active inflammation they have little or no application. Nevertheless, salicylates, phenylbutazone, oxyphenbutazone, indomethacin, the anthranilates and all those anti-inflammatory agents which also have analgesic properties may be helpful in such painful relatively inactive or grumbling chronic cases, though the corticosteroids, corticotrophin, tetracosactin, the gold salts, the antimalarials, penicillamine and the immunosuppressive agents, which have no analgesic action, are in general unhelpful.

Where one or a few joints are acutely inflamed, usually with an obvious effusion and increase of fluid in the affected joint, local aspiration and injection of hydrocortisone or other suitable corticosteroid into the joint will often benefit the local and sometimes the general condition also. This is partly due to reduction of the acute inflammation locally and partly the transient general effect of absorption of corticosteroid from the injection site. Such local therapy is very seldom complicated by infection or drug reaction, but it should only be used to control acute episodes of local disease activation occasionally when indicated and not repeatedly every few weeks. Temporary immobilization of such a joint in a plaster cast may also improve not only the local but the general condition also.

2. LOCAL PAIN DUE TO DESTRUCTIVE TISSUE CHANGES

Even when acute inflammatory changes have subsided in joint and periarticular tissues, pains may persist and be considerable and incapacitating. The effort to move contracted tissue and to bear weight, that is to use crippled joints, may cause considerable pain. In its control only those anti-inflammatory agents which have analgesic properties are helpful, the corticosteroids, for instance, in conservative dosage, only relieving pains when' it reduces local inflammation. The non-steroidal agents such as phenylbutazone, oxyphenbutazone and indomethacin and to a lesser extent the anthranilates and salicylates, are still helpful, along with the simple analgesics devoid of anti-inflammatory action; for example paracetamol, dextro-propoxyphene, codeine, dihydrocodeine and pentazocine. Potentially addictive drugs in a chronic condition with reasonable expectation of life such as rheumatoid arthritis should not be given unless there are complications or additional disorders which render the prognosis bad to within a few days or weeks. In such bad prognostic cases it is legitimate and ethical to prescribe first oral preparations of drugs such as diamorphine, morphine, papaveretum or dipipanone or suppositories such as proladone, and finally, if and when these means fail to control the pain, injections of physeptone, morphine, diamorphine or pethidine. Most rheumatoid patients, however, will never need such potentially addictive drugs and severe pain of crippling disease can often be controlled by intramuscular injections of dihydrocodeine (50–100 mg) or pentazocine (30–60 mg), when the usual oral preparations fail to make life tolerable for the sufferer. The addition of 10 mg of papaveretum to 500 mg of aspirin given as an effervescent tablet, 1 or 2 to be taken when pain is severe, is often extremely helpful and to those intolerant of aspirin, 1–1.5 g paracetamol as a suspension with 0.5–0.75 ml *tinct. opii*, a variation on the old fashioned 'mist. aspirin and nepenthe' theme may help considerably. Every patient, however, is an individual problem child as regards analgesia. Pain thresholds vary, and analgesics are often given unnecessarily when a few words of comfort and advice by physician, nurse, physiotherapist or friend would work equally well. The occupied mind needs less analgesia than one wide open to all painful stimuli, particularly at night when there are no distractions, and pain threshold has been shown (Huskisson and Hart, 1972) to be lowest in those rheumatoids confined to home who are unable to go out to work. As the ability to work depends in this disease essentially on pain, emphasis here must clearly be not only on activity and extent of rheumatoid disease, but also on the personality of the individual. Positive creative people (the *Typus robustus* of de Haas) need less analgesics than do what may be termed the *Typus supinus* of the unoccupied mind, who need considerable moral support and many daily analgesic tablets. Many 'positive' patients decline regular analgesics as they prefer to live with their pain, which they can tolerate, and which they prefer to tolerate without the assistance of analgesics which they find distasteful for psychological or pharmacological reasons, but others are less fortunate. In the final analysis most patients need analgesics repeatedly, some occasionally, a few seldom and a very few never. Whatever the official pharmacological half-life of the drug may be, the practical physician has to enquire from the patient the duration of action of any analgesic, the time of onset of action and any side effects. This is a part of the history-taking which is as essential and fundamental as the initial diagnostic case history. It throws a light not only on the drug's action but also on the personality of the consumer.

The final therapeutic attack on pain due to irreversible crippling disease is by surgery. Although synovectomy for inflammatory acute disease has been and is being widely performed, the long term results are still *sub-judice*. Where irreversible disease leaves gross dysfunction and pain there is, however, little argument except in detail as to what is done to which joint and when and by what technique. The Charnley and McKee–Farrer prostheses, arthrodesis of wrist and knee, and a number of other operations have wide application in the crippled rheumatoid joint, but a variety of operations performed on the rheumatoid knee, shoulder, ankle and elbow in the last decade are still under review.

3. SYSTEMIC ILLNESS IN RHEUMATOID ARTHRITIS

Pain caused by systemic illness is a much more complicated affair. It is a cocktail of aching all over the body and extremities, fever, tachycardia (palpitations), weakness (often partly due to anemia, which in turn is usually largely due to the active rheumatoid disease), unnatural fatigue and a number of other factors; it is a diffuse discomfort rather than a pain. Just as anemia is primarily due to dyshemopoiesis caused by the disease, so is the demoralizing systemic illness part of the prolonged active inflammatory disease. It can be reversed by corticosteroids, corticotrophin and tetracosactrin, but only at dose levels that produce unwanted Cushingoid effects. Some patients suffer little from systemic effects though greatly from articular symptoms, others largely from systemic and less from local disease. Therapy is essentially symptomatic. Adequate nutrition, blood transfusions, iron preparations by mouth and by injection and vitamins all help, but only remission, either natural or induced by prolonged therapy usually with anti-inflammatory agents such as gold salts, will reduce systemic pain and distress.

4. PSYCHIATRIC OVERTONES

It is an everyday experience of rheumatologists all over the world that anxiety and depression are a part of the clinical picture of long standing rheumatoid arthritis in a large percentage of patients at some time in the course of the disease. It is not generally accepted as a cause of the condition so much as a biproduct of the disorder. Symptomatic worsening or failure to improve on effective anti-rheumatic therapy may be due to these factors operating. Their presence may not be suspected as depressive or anxiety symptoms merge imperceptibly into the arthritic picture. Antidepressants have, therefore, a definite part to play in relieving distress, and pain may come under control with agents previously ineffective when anti-depressant agents are added. Anti-depressants fall very roughly into two main classes, the mildly stimulating such as imipramine, desipramine and protriptyline and the tranquillizing such as amitriptyline, nortriptyline, trimipramine and doxepin. Some patients benefit more with one, others with another. Amitriptyline or doxepin are in general more useful at night because of their sedative effect; Imipramine or protriptyline are more useful in the day. Both drugs take usually several days or 1–3 weeks for their beneficial effects in controlling depression to become apparent, but the tranquillizing action of amitriptyline is rapidly apparent. Scott (1969) found that the addition of imipramine under double-blind conditions improved the symptoms of 13 out of 22 rheumatoid patients, diminishing their daily pain as judged by their own statements. Nighttime is a bad time for depressed rheumatoid sufferers as pain interferes with sleep and anxiety and depression mounts as the hours pass and there is no distraction or escape from pain and the depression which so frequently accompanies it. From 5 a.m. onwards is the worst time for many rheumatoids and the stiffness and pain on rising are often merely the finale to a period of several hours of considerable distress. Anti-depressants may help here considerably. For the tense and anxious patient sedatives and tranquillizers — phenobarbitone, diazepam, meprobamate, amylobarbitone, chlordiazepoxide and occasionally the monoamineoxidase inhibitors — may help. These last, however, are in general best avoided in rheumatoid patients, who usually need several drugs daily and therefore run a greater risk of drug interactions. Amphetamine and combinations of amphetamine and amylobarbitone are useful in only a small number of depressed rheumatoids. Care must be taken lest too heavy sedation at night causes aggravation of morning pain and stiffness.

5. EXTRA-ARTICULAR MANIFESTATIONS

The acute pains of pericarditis and pleurisy in rheumatoid disease are usually mild and transient and do not call for more than simple analgesics. The pains of arterial occlusion in extremity, chest and abdomen may be slight, but if severe, may call for the most potent analgesics. Although Jaffe (1970) found penicillamine helpful for these patients, Huskisson and

Hart (1972b) in a small group of severely ill patients did not. Amputation of a digit or of a limb may be necessary; in such patients the prognosis is almost invariably grave. When vascular complications end the scene, narcotics may legitimately be used to ease pain and cloud consciousness if other drugs prove inadequate. The unpleasant sensations of peripheral rheumatoid neuropathy prove extremely difficult to control whatever combination of drugs is given, but the entrapment neuropathies, such as median nerve carpal tunnel compression, usually, though not invariably, respond to simple surgery but in a few unfortunate cases the pain of compression is followed and replaced by sensory changes resulting from the operation. Fractures and infections may occur readily in these patients whose bones are brittle and whose tissues are unduly liable to become affected. Atlanto–axial subluxation may cause symptoms of cord compression which may call for surgery, though rarely. Felty's syndrome should be mentioned in this connection for those patients with neutropenia and splenomegaly are very likely to suffer purulent complications in any part of the body. Splenectomy usually produces an immediate improvement, but Barnes (1971) and his co-workers have shown that a follow-up of these patients usually reveals considerable impairment of general health and not infrequently fresh episodes of infection which call for antibiotics and often for surgical drainage. The discomfort of the sicca (Sjögren's) syndrome (Shearn, 1972) is an added annoyance to a patient who, in addition to her painful arthritis, develops dry eyes, dry mouth and nose and occasionally a dry vaginal mucosa, with a remote risk of development of lymphoma.

6. THERAPEUTIC OVERTONES

All anti-inflammatory drugs taken by mouth may cause dyspepsia and peptic ulceration and this may add considerably to the patient's discomfort and cause difficulties in treatment. Antacids, milk feeds, and though rarely, surgery, may be necessary to control such symptoms. The anthranilates, mefenamic and flufenamic acids, may produce diarrhea, codeine constipation, indomethacin cerebral sensations, phenylbutazone and oxyphenbutazone blood disorders, the tricyclic depressants dry mouth, blurring of vision, difficulties with micturition and constipation because of their anticholinergic action, and so on. It is, however, the corticosteroids, cortico-trophin and tetracosactrin which produce the greatest change in almost all tissues of the body with some or all of the features of Cushing's disease. These drugs have been widely used in the past at too high dose levels and the dragging discomfort of being puffy and overweight, the lacerated and bruised fore-arms and shins and the acute pain of a crush fracture in an osteoporotic vertebra have to be added to the total discomfort of the patient's initial disease.

Conclusion

Pain in rheumatoid arthritis is therefore a mixture of many unpleasant stimuli; local, systemic, psychogenic and iatro-genic. Each facet of discomfort calls for separate and different forms of therapy, so that this is a disorder of many drugs and many possible drug interractions. While the therapeutic programme is kept as simple as possible, more than one or two drugs is usually necessary to control discomfort and make life tolerable and work or simple domestic duties possible. But it must be emphasized that we have found (Huskisson and Hart, 1972a) that the housebound patient has a lower pain threshold and needs more analgesic medication than the one at work with a job to do and an interest in it. The patient with an occupied mind needs much less medication than does what may be called the full-time sufferer.

Other inflammatory arthropathies

There are a large number of other inflammatory arthropathies (Huskisson and Hart, 1973) similar to rheumatoid arthritis but having other painful features peculiar to the condition, for instance the conjunctivitis and the non-specific urethritis of Brodie's (Reiter's) disease, the urethritis calling for tetracycline therapy. The arthropathy of ulcerative colitis should be men-tioned. It takes two forms, a peripheral joint involvement often occurring with an exacerbation of the colitis and a spinal and sacro-iliac involvement like that of ankylosing spondylitis. The colitis itself may cause considerable pain and discomfort calling for special medication such as corticosteroids by mouth and by retention enema, for sulphasalazine (salazopyrin) or surgery.

Where an inflammatory arthropathy is based on a treatable infection the necessary antibiotic is required—penicillin, cloxacillin or ampicillin, for instance—in gonococcal or septic arthropathy with local aspiration or drainage if needed. Psoriatic arthropathy may, like colitic arthropathy, present as a peripheral rheumatoid-like arthropathy or a central spondylitic one. In some cases a mixed picture is seen; in such cases treatment includes the measures described under ankylosing spondylitis and dermatological therapy for the psoriasis. Two conditions associated with an inflammatory arthropathy carry a more serious prognosis—systemic lupus erythematosus and polyarteritis nodosa. In both conditions pain arises from the same mixture of local, systemic and mental factors as is seen in severe rheumatoid disease. In both conditions corticosteroids usually have to be employed at some stage and often for some years and immunosuppressive agents may also be needed.

The ankylosing spondylarthropathies

The more one studies these disorders the greater the points of difference found between them and rheumatoid arthritis (Hart, 1968; 1971). The ankylosing spondylarthropathies include idiopathic ankylosing spondylitis and a similar clinical picture seen in some cases of Brodie's (Reiter's) disease, psoriatic arthropathy, the arthropathies associated with ulcerative colitis, Crohn's disease and Whipple's disease, Behçet's disease and a few late cases of male Still's disease. What is common to the pain patterns in this group of disorders is the diffuse spinal stiffening and the involvement of girdle joints, hip and shoulder, rather than peripheral and intermediate joints. In idiopathic ankylosing spondylitis, bony tenderness in pelvic and thoracic bones is common, and lytic areas occur in bones of pelvis and spine which may cause considerable pain and disability. Painful stiffness aggravated by immobility is the keynote of this group of disorders and symptoms are therefore worse at night and in the early morning, many patients rising from their beds two or three times a night to move about and limber up and so reduce the painful morning stiffness which is the major unpleasantness in this group of disorders. The patients with idiopathic ankylosing spondylitis, usually young males, are at their best when active and moving about and we have found their pain thresholds to be higher than in rheumatoid arthritis (Huskisson and Hart, 1972a). As a group these patients are more active, take less analgesic tablets and have less time off work than do rheumatoid arthritics. In the pre-war years therapeutic fashion was to restrict them in corsets and plaster jackets, emphasis being on spinal position rather than function. Happily this disastrous situation has been reversed and today these patients have exercise and exercises as a regular daily programme, emphasis being on bodily activity rather than rest. Although these patients share with rheumatoids painful nights and painfully stiff mornings, in most other respects their condition is a different one, graded rest being the rule in most rheumatoids, full activity short of fatigue and strain in the spondylitics in both idiopathic (primary) and secondary varieties. In the control of night pain and early morning stiffness the same anti-inflammatory drugs are used in the same dosage as in rheumatoid arthritis; Indomethacin by mouth or rectal suppository 75–100 mg or prednisolone or prednisone 5 mg by mouth on retiring. In the control of symptoms in the day phenylbutazone or oxyphenbutazone 100–400 mg in divided dose by mouth is indicated at the lowest effective dose or indomethacin 25–100 mg with food in divided doses, also at the lowest effective level. Rarely is it necessary to use corticosteroids, corticotrophins or tetracosactrin in these cases, but any of the other anti-inflammatory or analgesic agents listed above in the treatment of rheumatoid arthritis may be helpful in milder cases, given as required in the day. The use of these drugs by day or night is not only to make life more painfree for the sufferer but also to encourage better and more free function and greater mobility by day and less morning stiffness with more restful and less painful nights. Salicylates are less helpful in the spondylarthropathies than in rheumatoid arthritis and in general analgesics much less effective than anti-inflammatory agents such as phenylbutazone, oxyphenbutazone and indomethacin. Gold salts and the antimalarials have not been found to be effective in this group of disorders, but deep x-ray therapy locally applied to the affected areas of the spine and to the sacro-iliac joints in particular in conservative skin dosage of around 1000 r has been found to be helpful in reducing painful stiffness and local tenderness, though at the price of increasing the risk of acute leukemia in these patients, a risk which though present may have been over-emphasized in the past (Sinclair, 1971). Although the essence of therapy in the ankylosing spondyl arthropathies is full mobility short of fatigue and strain under cover of suitable therapeutic agents, sudden localized exacerbation of painful symptoms may be the result of local injury, such as strain, subluxation or fracture, for the stiffened ankylosed spine is overprone to such traumatic lesions. In such cases rest and analgesics are indicated with splintage and occasionally surgical fusion of the hypermobile area. Between two fixed immobile segments of the spine such an area of painful hyper-mobility may occur, a painful false joint or pseudoarthrosis which may similarly need rest, immobility and occasionally surgical fusion. Local bony tenderness in the spondylartho-pathies may be found most commonly in ischial tuberosities, crests of pelvis, symphysis pubis, sternum, ribs anteriorly, sterno-clavicular joints, the heels and various parts of the spine. Simple analgesics or simple local measures, such as cushions for the ischial tuberosities or soft insoles or soft shoes for the heels, are all that is usually indicated as these symptoms subside spontaneously in most cases in a few months, but local deep x-ray therapy in low dosage 200–400 r may relieve symptoms in those very few cases not controlled by simple measures. This local form of deep x-ray therapy is, however, only very rarely necessary. One further painful aspect may be mentioned and that is iridocyclitis, which occurs commonly in the idiopathic variety in around 20–25% of cases, not un-commonly in Reiter's disease and occasionally in the other variants. Atropine-like drugs and local corticosteroids are indicated here. Aortic insufficiency occurs as part of the idio-pathic disease in about 1–2% of cases and may be associated with heart failure or infective endocarditis, which in turn calls for appropriate therapeutic measures.

Finally, as most discomfort in ankylosing spondylitis is experienced at night, what of the patient's sleeping conditions? A firm hard mattress is usually preferred, often with boards underneath. Air inflated mattresses of the sort used on bathing beaches may give much relief, and gentle electrical agitation of the bed may ease painful symptoms at night (Hart, 1973) and many patients sleep better on ships or trains than at home in bed. These patients, particularly the young male idiopathic spondylitics, suffer less depression and emotional overtones than do the rheumatoids and their usually normal peripheral joints enable them to lead more normal lives. Affected hips, however, often cause considerable pain and crippling and the Charnley and McKee–Farrer operations would appear to offer more than previous orthopedic operations on the hip, though adequate follow-up information over a post-operative period of several years is not as yet forthcoming in this group of patients.

Gout

In acute gout the patient suffers agony. The affected area is acutely inflamed, tense, swollen and tender. There are no overtones of chronic anxiety or depression, merely frustration and annoyance sometimes pushed to the point of rage. In the vast majority of cases the attack is short lived and rapidly controlled by effective agents, colchicine, phenylbutazone, oxyphenbutazone or indomethacin. The essence of rapid control of the acute attack lies in education of the sufferer in the early treatment of the acute attack with the appropriate drug, for the longer the acute attack is allowed to continue untreated, the longer it takes to come under control. The gouty subject is therefore instructed to take the drug which has proved effective and non-toxic previously at the first definite signs of the acute attack. Some patients prefer the old remedy colchicine, taking initially 1 mg (two tablets of 0.5 mg) then $\frac{1}{2}$ mg hourly for 4–5 doses reducing thereafter to $\frac{1}{2}$ mg 2–3 hourly until the attack is controlled, a total of 6 mg (12 tablets) has been taken or diarrhea has developed, dosage being then reduced to $\frac{1}{2}$ mg 3 or 4 times a day and gradually discontinued over the next 3–4 days. The most common toxic effect is diarrhea and for this reason most patients prefer phenylbutazone or oxyphenbutazone 600–800 mg in divided dosage on day one, dosage being reduced by 100 mg daily. Phenylbutazone may be given by intramuscular injection and phenylbutazone and oxyphenbutazone in suppository form if these drugs are poorly tolerated by mouth. Quicker in action is indomethacin, which is given in 25–50 mg doses with food 3 or 4 times a day or perhaps

more effectively as a 75–100 mg dosage with food at night or
as a suppository (100 mg) on retiring, followed by 25 mg 3 or 4
times a day with food, dosage being gradually reduced as the
attack comes under control. These measures usually abate the
attack within 24–72 hours and it is only when they fail, which
is rarely, that treatment of the pain of chronic, or, to be more
precise, persistent acute gout has to be considered. Here, if
partially effective, the non-steroidal drugs mentioned above
can be continued in conjunction with corticosteroids or corticotrophin or tetracosactrin but in most cases the last named are
given alone; prednisolone or prednisone 40–50 mg by mouth
daily, dosage being reduced as rapidly as possible as the attack
comes under control, or corticotrophin gel 60 units by intramuscular injection, dosage again being reduced by 5–10 units
daily; or tetracosactrin 0.6–1 ml by intramuscular injection
reducing by 0.1 ml daily. Only rarely is it necessary to resort
to these agents which are best avoided because of their steroidal
overtones. Occasionally aspiration of an acutely inflamed
gouty joint with injection of hydrocortisone or other suitable
preparation intra-articularly proves helpful. In general, however, prevention of gout today with allopurinol, probenecid,
ethebenecid or sulphinpyrazone has replaced anti-inflammatory therapy of prolonged gouty attacks which are now only
rarely seen, and local applications to the affected inflamed joint
are things of the past.

Polymyalgia rheumatica and giant cell arteritis

Polymyalgia rheumatica is perhaps a less satisfactory title than
polymyalgia arteritica (Hamrin *et al.*, 1964) for it is often, if
not usually, merely an articular phase of giant cell (temporal
or cranial) arteritis. In a subject past middle age, usually
female and over 60 years of age, the characteristic symptoms
are marked painful stiffness in the early mornings in shoulder
and hip girdles, almost invariably accompanied by a markedly
elevated erythrocyte sedimentation rate, usually over 60 mm
in 1 hour. The patients often have obvious evidence of
degenerative joint disease and have usually been incapacitated in great degree for many weeks or months, but the
high sedimentation rate, presence of girdle joint early morning painful stiffness and absence of signs of rheumatoid

arthritis in the peripheral and intermediate joints points strongly to polymyalgia rheumatica. Response to small doses of corticosteroids, such as 2.5 mg of prednisolone four times daily is usually dramatic, and dosage thereafter has to be very slowly and gradually reduced over periods of many months as the disease does not usually subside until many months or 3–5 years have elapsed. Dosage reduction must therefore be according to symptomatic control and normalization of sedimentation rate and too rapid reduction of corticosteroid dosage will be followed by a rapid return of symptoms. In control of giant cell arteritis when cranial or cerebral vessels are affected, dosage should be higher because of the risk of blindness from involvement of the central retinal arteries, 40–50 mg of prednisolone daily in divided dosage, subsequent reduction being effected according to symptomatology and sedimentation rate levels. The risk of blindness is present also in polymyalgia rheumatica but is much less. Other anti-inflammatory agents may produce some symptomatic ease, but as they are less effective than the corticosteroids, which remain the most effective anti-inflammatory agents we have, they are unlikely to prevent fresh arterial occlusion, the most vulnerable area being the eye. Early correct diagnosis and early therapy will therefore not only produce rapid relief of symptoms in both disorders, but also prevent blindness.

Osteoarthrosis

We all grow old and our cartilages age steadily and show increasing evidence of degenerative change from the early twenties onwards. X-rays of most of us past middle age show degenerative change, but one is only allowed to use the term osteoarthrosis when these changes cause symptoms: pain, stiffness, restricted range of movement, weakness and some disability. Such painful changes are seen more often in certain families: grandmother, mother and daughter may all show similar changes but in different degree, for instance, in the terminal interphalangeal joints of the fingers (Heberden's nodes). Osteoarthrotic changes associated with pain and with other symptoms may occur in (a) diffuse form affecting terminal interphalangeal joints, thumb bases and possibly neck, lumbar spine, knees, hips and acromio-clavicular joints, the generalized osteoarthrosis of Kellgren and Moore (1952), particularly in females about the time of the menopause or shortly afterwards, and particularly if parents were similarly affected: (b) in scattered patchy distribution in these same areas in older patients of either sex: (c) in joints previously traumatized where local damage, hemarthrosis or subluxation has occurred: (d) more rarely, where there is a prior defect in pain appreciation, unnatural tissue fragility, abnormal nutritional factors or congenital defect (Hart, 1973). The march of events varies according to the individual case and the local factors operating, but essentially degenerative changes with friability and fragmentation of cartilage, thickening and eburnation of adjacent bone with narrowing of joint space and redistribution of bone alignment is evident, a variable degree of synovial proliferation and vascular change and a very variable amount of pain and stiffness and disability ranging from slight to extreme. Symptoms may have little apparent relation to structural change as evidenced by clinical or radiological features and gross changes may be accompanied by little or no pain in one patient and considerable discomfort and disability in another. Although personality, pain threshold and other factors play a part, there is no doubt that considerable differences in pain production do occur in similar lesions. Heberden's nodes, for instance the bony bossed osteoarthritic terminal interphalangeal joints of the fingers, are usually unsightly and awkward to use, but are seldom painful when fully developed. In their early stages, however, they may show all the cardinal signs of inflammation, the terminal joint being red, tense, tender to touch and painful to move. These 'hot' Heberden's nodes would appear to be caused by release of hyaluronic acid into the surrounding tissues from the degenerating cartilage, so setting up an acutely painful inflammatory reaction. A second cause of pain in more advanced osteoarthrotic joints is injury, small subluxations and bruising causing local pain. In joints such as the knees a sudden exacerbation of pain is accompanied by swelling in the joint, aspiration of bloodstained fluid confirming the traumatic nature of the exacerbation in many cases. The quality and nature of the symptoms and the factors which ease or aggravate osteoarthrotic joints will differ in different individuals but even more in different joints, the pain syndromes in osteoarthrosis of cervical and lumbar spines, hips, knees, thumb bases, fingers and acromio-clavicular joints responding to different forms of therapy. Chronic pain due to osteoarthrosis can be controlled largely or in part by five different approaches:

(1) Simple analgesics and anti-inflammatory agents with analgesic properties.

(2) Rest, splintage and supports.

(3) Other physical measures; exercises, heat and cold, active and passive movements, hydrotherapy, local applications and injections.

(4) Surgery.

(5) Sedatives and psychotropic agents.

(1) SIMPLE ANALGESICS AND ANTI-INFLAMMATORY AGENTS

These may be used to help control pain in any osteoarthrotic area, but they are often of slight help except when pain is mild. Nevertheless, any or all of the analgesics and anti-inflammatory agents mentioned previously may be tried and usually suffice to make life bearable for many months or years. In osteoarthrosis of the hip, for instance, Wanka and Dixon (1964) found indomethacin helpful, and phenylbutazone or oxyphenbutazone will often ease pains considerably, as may salicylates, the anthranilates and simple analgesics such as paracetamol, dextropropoxyphene, codeine, dihydrocodeine or pentazocine. In many cases, particularly in patients with chronic and recurring pain of osteoarthrosis of fingers, thumb bases and cervical and lumbar spines, analgesics are of relatively little help unless accompanied by physical measures also. Local injections of anesthetic or steroid agents have little and limited application. The virtue of phenylbutazone and oxyphenbutazone lies in their even and long-continued action, but they are often inadequate in controlling pain effectively and long continued use carries the risk of aplastic anemia.

(2) REST, SPLINTAGE AND SUPPORTS

The very painful osteoarthrotic joint, wherever it is in the body, must be rested, for use will aggravate the discomfort and maintain the disability. An acutely painful cervical spondylosis must be rested in bed with supporting pillows. often with a plaster shell or collar and neck traction if compression pain causes reference down the arms, a lighter plastic collar being worn as symptoms ease and the patient is able to resume activities out of bed. The very painful knee or lumbar spine must also be rested until acute symptoms abate.

(3) OTHER PHYSICAL AGENTS — EXERCISES, ETC.

Excessive rest also causes pain in an osteoarthrotic joint, exercise and change of position relieving it. This is particularly seen in knee and hip, where prolonged sitting with these joints in flexion to 90° or more will cause considerable discomfort, particularly after 30–40 minutes immobility, relief being rapidly obtained by extending the leg and rising and walking about. This pain of immobility is seen in other joints on occasion, particularly when held for prolonged intervals in unnatural positions, but the fixed-flexion pain is most commonly seen in the knee after prolonged sitting at desk, table or in an automobile. Exercise and exercises are essential to prevent contraction of the various joint capsules, which in osteoarthrosis prevent movements initially because of pain, this in turn leading to further limitation of movement and contraction. The use of sticks, crutches and various devices in home, office and automobile may reduce pains considerably and lead to better function. Heat and cold and a variety of forms of physiotherapy merely aid this programme of exercise, prevention of deformities and contractions and maintenance of muscle integrity. Exercises in warm water, i.e. assisted movements in a warm medium, are often very effective not only in increasing mobility but in easing pain. This excellent form of therapy was used by the Romans in the heavy salt-water baths found still in certain spas such as Droitwich in this country and the application of warm mud (fango) or clay to painful osteoarthrotic joints is still popular throughout Europe.

(4) SURGERY

It is the chronic recurrent pain of osteoarthrosis which demoralizes the patient, prevents normal function and cripples him. The patient with a painless but grossly distorted neuropathic (Charcot) joint hobbles through life comparatively cheerfully compared with the painful arthritic sufferer, who cannot move without pain. Analgesics, however effective, and physical measures, however well administered, will only ease the pain load but will not cure it. The pain arises from the capsule and tendon insertions in particular, but also from other components in joint and surrounding structures and these pains are often referred to points some distance from the joint so that the patient with severe osteoarthrosis of the hip asks for treatment for the knee below it. Where all painful structures are removed, as in the Charnley or McKee–Farrer operations of the hip, and a prosthesis replaces the affected joint, the immediate relief of pain and the rapidity of convalescence as a result is remarkable. As Charnley (1971) himself comments, not only is physiotherapy not usually needed, but the patient often has to be restrained from doing too much. This happy state of affairs results essentially from the fact that the pain-producing tissues have been completely ablated. Arthrodesis does the same for the knee, replacing painful mobile structures by a fixed painless long bone. Removal of the acromion process or the carpal bone may relieve pain in shoulder or thumb-base but the complete hip prosthetic replacement is to date the most dramatic demonstration of the effect of pain relief on function in orthopedic surgery.

(5) SEDATIVES AND PSYCHOTROPIC AGENTS

Psychic overtones are perhaps less common in patients with osteoarthrosis than in patients with rheumatoid arthritis as they are not systemically ill, as are the latter. Nevertheless, the unremitting and persistent nature of the discomfort and the thwarting nature of the disability which prevents the normal enjoyment of the day's activities at work and at home brings its spiritual overtones and angry resentment, irritation, anxiety, depression and even despair may result. Sedatives and anti-depressants are, however, less likely to be needed in osteoarthrotic sufferers than in rheumatoids, but much physio and supportive therapy given to these patients works as much through mood as through matter. It is indeed supportive sympathetic therapy. Somebody is caring and giving a helpful hand. The danger here lies in the patient becoming too reliant on others and becoming too passive in her approach to her own disorder.

Paget's disease of bone

Paget's disease of bone is a chronic disorder of unknown etiology characterized by considerable changes in shape and texture of bone with typical radiological changes. Microscopically there is replacement of normal structure by bone which is morphologically and chemically abnormal. There are abnormal irregular trabecular surfaces with an increase in osteoblastic osteoid production and osteoclastic resorption, the bone being considerably more vascular than normal with an increase in fibroblasts and fibrous tissue. The normal compact cortical bone is gradually replaced by a cancellous type of bone structure which results in an abnormally thick cortex. The condition affects males more often than females and is most common after middle age. Many cases are symptomless and are discovered accidentally on routine radiology or by chance discovery of raised figures of plasma alkaline phosphatase, but in some there is considerable discomfort. Pain is sometimes the presenting symptom, a dull deep persistent nagging ache, increasing in intensity with time but sometimes switching off, the condition becoming largely or completely painless, even though biochemically and radiologically it appears to be unchanged or progressing. Enlargement of the skull may be associated with headaches and deafness, and deformities of extremities with pains in the arm or, more commonly, the leg. Involvement of pelvis and spine may cause backache and postural deformities. Fractures occur readily and sarcomatous change may be accompanied by appearance of, or considerable increase in, pain. Hypercalcuria may be associated with pains of renal calculus formation and excretion, and hypercalcemia, aggravated by immobility, as after a fracture in a bone affected by the disease, may cause nausea, vomiting, dehydration and even death. If sudden pain occurs in a patient with Paget's disease, the physician should suspect either a fracture or malignant change.

Pain in Paget's disease therefore ranges from none whatsoever to the agony of an osteogenic sarcoma calling for amputation and/or deep x-ray therapy. Simple analgesics are all that is necessary in some cases, but pain may be so intense, particularly in sarcomatous cases, that narcotics are necessary. Sodium fluoride (Avioli and Berman, 1968) has been used in high dosage to reduce serum alkaline phosphatase and urine hydroxyproline levels and this has been accompanied by relief from pain. High levels of fluoride are, however, potentially toxic and might possibly lead to skeletal fluosis. Large infusions of glucagon (Condon, 1971) have also resulted in relief of bone pain and reduction in bone resorption, but it has been the development of calcitonin (Bijvoet and Jansen, 1967) which perhaps promises to be the most helpful form of therapy in selected painful progressive cases. It is a polypeptide hormone secreted by the parafollicular cells of the thyroid gland in mammals and though porcine, human and salmon calcitonin has been used in certain studies only the porcine variety is commercially available. Calcitonin inhibits bone resorption and lowers both serum and urinary calcium concentrations; the reduction in bone turnover has been accompanied by relief of pain in long term studies (Bell *et al.*, 1970; Haddad *et al.*, 1970). Treatment has to be continued indefinitely, for biochemical parameters revert and pain returns on withdrawal of the drug. Calcitonin is given daily by intramuscular or subcutaneous injection, a total of 0.5–2.0 MRC units per kg per day initially twice a day, morning and evening. In patients with a history of allergy, sensitivity tests should be done before therapy is started and plasma calcium levels should be monitored repeatedly. It is at present an expensive form of therapy, and as in the vast majority of cases pain is slight or non-existent, need only be employed in a minority of cases. Pain due to bone hyperemia, bone deformity and nerve compression have been relieved within a few weeks of starting treatment (Haddad *et al.*, 1970).

Chronic backache
One of the commonest pains in patients in general practice is backache. The causes are many (Hart, 1973) and various and the first step in understanding backache is to identify the nature and distribution of the receptor systems and their different pathways in the deep tissues of the back, whose irritation may give rise to this common complaint (Wyke, 1967; 1973). This author suggests that backache may arise by one or more of the following mechanisms:

    1. Primary backache arising from (a) nerve endings in

capsules of apophyseal joints, (b) spinal ligaments, (c) vertebral periosteum and attached fasciae and tendons, (d) dura mater and epidural adipose tissue, (e) walls of arterioles supplying vertebral cancellous bone and (f) walls of epidural and paravertebral veins.

2. Secondary backache from pain afferent fibers in dorsal nerve roots and their branches serving the receptor systems noted above.

3. Reflex backache, owing to reflex spasm of paravertebral musculature causing irritation of perivascular nerve plexuses in the walls of intramuscular arterioles.

4. Referred backache from irritation of pain receptor systems distributed through visceral tissues segmentally innervated from dorsal spine nerve roots.

The commonest conditions associated with or actually causing chronic backache are the following:

1. Traumatic and degenerative: faulty posture; obesity and strain; injury with fracture or subluxation and secondary degenerative changes; disc degeneration and prolapse; spondylolisthesis.

2. Metabolic states: osteoporosis; osteomalacia; hyperparathyroidism and Paget's disease.

3. Inflammatory arthropathies: ankylosing spondylitis; secondary spondylitis and more rarely polymyalgia rheumatica; rheumatoid arthritis; systemic lupus erythematosus and polyarteritis nodosa.

4. Infective arthropathies: tuberculosis; brucellosis; typhoid and paratyphoid fever; osteomyelitis, leptospirosis icterohemorrhagica.

5. Psychogenic: hysteria; anxiety states; depression; malingering; compensation neurosis.

6. Spinal tumors; primary and secondary.

7. Referred from intrathoracic disease: aortic aneurysm; carcinoma of the bronchus and esophagus.

8. Referred from abdominal disease: carcinoma of the pancreas, chronic pancreatitis; ascites; pyelonephritis; carcinoma of the kidney.

9. Referred from pelvic disease: tuberculous endometritis; prostatitis; carcinoma of the prostate.

This by no means completes the list, but setting out the

main causative or associated conditions does at least reveal the complexity of the subject and the varied therapeutic approaches indicated. Backache and its treatment covers much of medicine and of orthopedics. Where surgical cure is possible or drug therapy curative the approach is straightforward, but otherwise the general principles are sometimes in sharp contrast. For instance in tuberculous disease or fractures of spine and recent crush fractures in an osteoporotic spine rest is essential, if necessary in a plaster cast. The same treatment applied to a patient with ankylosing spondylitis would cripple him, for here mobility, exercise and exercises are all important under cover of analgesics or anti-inflammatory agents in most cases. Even in ankylosing spondylitis rest and even spinal fusion may be necessary when painful areas of hypermobility between fixed painless segments of the vertebral column occur. The treatment of the commonest causes, back strain and degenerative and disc disease, lies essentially in conservative and common sense physical measures such as adjustment of chairs, beds and car seats to avoid bad posture, supportive jackets occasionally, and exercises and graded rest with analgesic drugs as and if required. When one looks, however, at the potential pain producing areas in the spine and the many conditions which may affect them, treatment becomes essentially empirical. Even where infection may be completely eradicated, as in tuberculous or brucellar infection or in leptospirosis icterohemorrhagica, persistent degenerative and destructive sequelae may persist in chronic painful form. In primary or secondary osteoarthrosis, manipulative therapy of the spine is often effective in relieving pain, sometimes dramatically so. It is often ineffective, however, and may make pains worse if applied in the wrong way at the wrong time. For a patient with a persisting and demoralizing backache due, for instance, to a prolapsed intervertebral disc, any treatment is welcome if it offers hope of cure, and manipulation may ease symptoms in many cases as much through psyche as through soma. Where backache is essentially psychogenic in origin or is psychologically maintained, manipulation often proves helpful, but usually not curative, for the basic underlying mental attitude remains unchanged, whether it is based on unhappiness in the home or a pending claim for compensation. The popularity in the past and in the present for massage, another mode of laying on of healing hands, depends greatly on the soothing and sympathetic approach in those many cases where pain has a spiritual or psychic background rather than an organic one. Even given an obvious organic cause such treatment though palliative is often very popular as it soothes even if it does not cure and makes the patient feel he is not alone in his suffering and his struggle toward a cure. Heat applied to a painful area in a spine will often ease symptoms considerably whatever the cause. Traction is more effective in compression syndromes in the neck, as in cervical disc lesions, where it may produce considerable relief. Heat soothes most pains and aches whatever the cause or causes but a lasting relief after traction and manipulation usually suggests a mechanical basis.

In the control of chronic pain in the back, therefore, the problem is almost as large as medicine and orthopedics. Not only is the spine a highly elaborate construction held for most of the day in odd and unnatural positions in civilized man, but it might almost have been designed as a model for the experimental production of pain. Subject it to the great variety of traumatic and pathological processes found in medicine and it is no small wonder that we all suffer backache at some time in our lives and often for considerable periods.

To summarize in this difficult field; the practical points in pain relief, whatever the cause of the backache, are as follows:

1. Rest or activity. The first decision is to either rest the patient completely, as in an acute disc protrusion, a crush fracture or an acute Pott's disease; to rest him partially with periods of exercise, as in osteoporosis and osteomalacia; or as little as possible, as in ankylosing spondylitis. Even in these disorders the programme of rest has to be tailored to the particular patient. Complete restriction in plaster casts may be called for in some cases, but less commonly than in the past.

2. Exercises. After the initial acute painful phase of a severe backache when, whatever the cause, rest has to be the initial approach, a period of rehabilitation and exercise is required to restore function and as much mobility as is reasonably possible. Local heat and exercises in warm water (balneotherapy) are often very helpful in this program of rehabilitation. In stiffening conditions such as the ankylosing

spondylarthropathies exercises are indicated from the start except in a small number of very acute cases, or cases with hypermobile areas in the spine or with spinal injuries. Postural and breathing exercises are a part of this program and the patient must be instructed to persist with his own exercises in most cases and to be told clearly what to do and what not to do in the future; that is:

3. Indoctrination in how to lead his future life in relation to his chronic back condition. This involves a study of the car in which he drives, the chairs in which he sits, the bed in which he lies and the office desk or work-bench at which he earns his living. Certain beds designed to prevent bed sores have proved useful in chronic backaches of different sorts, as for instance inflatable mattresses or cushions or pads filled with expanded polystyrene granules, which shift to mould easily to the patient's body, spreading pressure more evenly over a larger area of the surface (Hill, 1973). Walking sticks, supports or crutches may have to be selected and their use explained in some cases at some period in the program of rehabilitation.

4. Attention to general physical and mental health. Diet: many overweight patients have backaches which are improved by weight reduction and factors such as anemia and depression may be present and may need attention.

5. Specific therapy if indicated, for infective conditions such as tuberculosis, brucellosis, pyemic conditions or syphilis (today extremely rare as a cause of backache) or neoplastic conditions such as Hodgkin's disease, myeloma or malignant disease of the spine, primary or secondary.

6. Simple analgesic or anti-inflammatory drugs, the selection and timing depending on the nature of the backache.

7. Narcotic analgesics when pain is severe and outlook grave.

8. Psychotropic drugs or psychotherapy in selected cases. In all cases of chronic backache, however, some moral and mental support is required by the patient from physician, nurse, physiotherapist and those around him.

9. Surgery in selected cases, e.g. removal of prolapsed disc pressing on nervous tissue, spinal fusion, removal of malignant or benign growths (e.g. osteoid osteoma).

10. Radiotherapy or cytotoxic therapy may be indicated in some cases.

11. Extradural corticosteroid injections. These are of use in the management of lumbar nerve root compression. They are discussed in Chapter 6.

Whatever the cause of the backache it is likely that at least four of the above eleven forms of therapy will be needed and in many cases more. Yet looking at random into the current textbooks of rheumatology on my shelves backache appears as a title only in the index of two of them.

HEAT AND COLD

Throughout rheumatology, in all the different less severe clinical conditions heat in some form usually gives some measure of relief. Licht (1968) states that heat produces relief of pain, muscle relaxation, sedation and increased local circulation whether given as moist heat with saturated moist warm air, as wet towels or immersion, or as dry heat in different forms. The choice of methods depends, as Licht observes, either on the training and experience of the physician or on empiricism. He gives for 1968, when his book was published, the relative popularity in the United States as follows: for muscle spasm hot moist packs, for arthritis of the hands paraffin baths, for low back pain diathermy, for arthritis and pains in the neck an incandescent lamp. The dosage, he continues, is a matter of opinion rather than fact and opinion also varies greatly on method, source of heat and the duration and frequency of therapy. Heat, if it helps, needs to be given at least once daily and if great relief is obtained probably twice. Licht considers that with heat treatment, which in general is applied in increasing duration up to 30 minutes at a time, it should be comfortable throughout its application and at the end of therapy the skin should be pink and warm, not red and hot and this deep pink color should disappear in about twenty minutes after completion of therapy. Such treatment can be overdone and produce skin lesions and aggravation of the condition it was meant to help. The period just after heat has been applied would appear to be a suitable time for the patient to exercise the affected part, and we have found exercises in a warm deep pool perhaps the most helpful of all methods in relieving pain and facilitating movements in many rheumatological conditions: the deep warm pool is popular with nine out of every ten of our patients who have tried this form of therapy. On return home the best time for exercises is after a warm bath or shower and much relief from pain and increase in function can be achieved by the patient with simple home measures. The hand in rheumatoid arthritis in my experience is often aggravated by dry heat but improves after warm soaks or wax. But there is no magic virtue in any particular form or application of heat and patients will continue or stop home treatment depending on the therapeutic response. A hot bath in the home is usually more helpful for the rheumatoid polyarthritic than any other form of home therapy as she has less total pain, relaxes, moves better subsequently and in her exercises afterwards can attain and maintain a greater range of joint movement in all joints than previously. Hot mud (fango) is still popular in many spas in Europe and is given mostly for degenerative conditions. Cold has usually a worsening or aggravating effect on inflamed joints but application of cold packs to the affected limb may in some cases lead to an 'afterglow' which the patient finds beneficial and which enables her to perform her exercises more effectively. Tissues may be cooled by convection, evaporation by spraying with volatile liquids or by conduction, applying solids, liquids or gases but usually ice, at temperatures lower than that of the skin. Pain may subsequently be relieved and range of movements increased, but not in all cases. Many patients derive little benefit and in some a worsening occurs. Whether heat or cold is used, pain relief is transient only, the aim being to rehabilitate the patient and improve function rather than to achieve lasting pain relief. One of the most ancient forms of applied heat can be seen in the home treatment of osteoarthrosis in the elderly in some Mediterranean countries, grandfather or grandmother being taken to the beach in the morning, buried in the hot sand with a parasol over his or her head and a flask of wine or water placed alongside, the patient being dug up in the evening, by now gently relaxed and in less pain, to be taken home to have supper.

ANALGESIC DRUGS
So far in this chapter the approach to the relief and control of pain has been the clinical one, that is from the anguished patient

in pain to the drug. Let us reverse this approach and look at pain relief in terms of drug reaction and effect. What analgesic and anti-inflammatory analgesic substances are best for which conditions? In this different physicians and their patients have different views: what follows is therefore personal but based on many drug trials and many patients' statements over many years. Only essentially non-addictive drugs will be considered.

Aspirin

Aspirin in its various forms has completely replaced sodium salicylate as an effective reliever of pain. It is rapidly absorbed, is quickly effective within 15–25 minutes but lasts only 1–4 hours depending on the intensity and quality of the underlying painful condition. In full dosage of 5 g daily or more, taken 3–4 hourly with food, it is demonstrably anti-inflammatory in rheumatoid patients, but it is effective as an analgesic in lower dosage (Boardman and Hart, 1967). It has a complex and varied action and may inter-react with other drugs. In gout, for instance, it tends to elevate serum urate levels in small doses and lowers them in high dosage and it also interferes with the uricosuric action of probenecid. The conditions in which it is most effective are the inflammatory arthropathies, such as rheumatoid arthritis. It is helpful in degenerative and traumatic conditions but is of little help in acute gout. In ankylosing spondylitis it usually helps only the mildest cases, but is useful to control traumatic painful episodes. Its main side effects are gastro-intestinal irritation, nausea and tinnitus. The elderly tolerate it less well than the young. It remains an essential drug for most arthritic patients, and the soluble forms are preferred by the majority of patients. Good formulation is essential. The fact that different preparations contain the same amount of drug per tablet does not mean that all are equally effective.

The pyrazoles

Phenylbutazone and oxyphenbutazone exert a prolonged relatively even analgesic and anti-inflammatory action and have proved their worth in osteoarthrosis, ankylosing spondylitis and the inflammatory arthropathies. They are useful also in a wide range of painful conditions of bone and joint, even in malignancy if pain is not extreme. They may be given by mouth or suppository and phenylbutazone by intramuscular injection. Although a wide range of toxic effects have been reported it is the hematological complications of aplasia, neutropenia and thrombocytopenia that are, though rare, the most dangerous. Water loading in elderly cardiacs may occur. Clinical effect is often not apparent until several hours or a day or more after starting therapy. It displaces anticoagulants such as Warfarin from binding sites on serum proteins and should never be given with oral anticoagulants.

Indomethacin

This has a shorter action than phenylbutazone, clinical effects being noted within two hours, passing off in 6–12 hours depending on dosage. It may be given by mouth or suppository. It is effective in relieving pain in gout, ankylosing spondylitis, rheumatoid arthritis, Reiter's disease and other inflammatory arthropathies, also in osteoarthrosis. As it is excreted largely in the urine, renal function should be known to be normal before administration of the drug. Headaches and various unpleasant cerebral sensations are manifestations of too high blood levels, as tinnitus and deafness are with salicylate overdosage. Gastro-intestinal irritation may occur, as it may with all effective anti-inflammatory analgesic agents.

The anthranilates

Anthranilates — mefenamic and flufenamic acids — are anti-inflammatory analgesic agents which I would place at a lower effective level than the pyrazoles or indomethacin. They may be helpful in inflammatory arthropathies where other agents are poorly tolerated and may help also in degenerative painful conditions, their main side effect being diarrhea.

Ibuprofen

This is an analgesic with anti-inflammatory properties demonstrable in experimental animal models but only rarely in man. It is in general well tolerated and individual patients derive considerable benefit, but in general it is a relatively mild analgesic.

Paracetamol

This is a mild antipyretic and analgesic agent, but it has no anti-inflammatory action. Its use is therefore in mild degenerative painful conditions and in rheumatoid arthritics with pain of mild nature based not on acute inflammatory changes but on residual damage of articular tissues. It is usually well-tolerated by the gastro-intestinal tract and though similar chemically to phenacetin has relatively little against it as regards renal toxicity.

Phenacetin

Use of this substance has been largely discontinued because of its ability to produce enterogenous cyanosis (sulphemoglobinemia and methemoglobinemia) and its possible renal toxicity when used in compound analgesic tablets. Although never today used alone, it is present in many compound analgesic tablets which may still be purchased without prescription in Britain.

Amidopyrine

This also has been very largely given up in Britain as an analgesic because of the risks of its causing agranulocytosis. It is an effective analgesic, however, and is still largely used in certain countries in Europe, but it was removed from the British Pharmaceutical Codex some 35 years ago.

Dihydrocodeine

This is a mild analgesic with slight tranquillizing properties. It has no anti-inflammatory effect and is slightly constipating. Taken in doses of 60 mg (two tablets) it is often more effective than paracetamol or dextropropoxyphene, particularly at night. Given by intramuscular injection in doses of 50–100 mg it is effective in a wide range of painful conditions ranging from rheumatoid arthritis and osteoarthrosis to metastatic malignant disease. Here it has the virtue of being known only as an 'antirheumatic' analgesic agent, so that the sufferer, who may not know the true malignant nature of her condition, will accept it the more readily. It is weakly addictive and is now controlled under the Misuse of Drugs Regulations.

Codeine phosphate

This is a weak analgesic with constipating properties. It is in my experience more effective in controlling mild diarrhea than pain.

Dextropropoxyphene

Another well-tolerated weak analgesic without anti-inflammatory properties. A sustained action tablet is available.

Pentazocine

This is an analgesic which, like dihydrocodeine, is only very weakly addictive and is therefore not on the addictive drug schedule. It is a weak analgesic given by mouth in doses of 25–75 mg but is more effective by subcutaneous or intramuscular injection, 30–60 mg.

Benorylate

This recently produced compound breaks down to paracetamol and salicylate in the intestinal tract. It may be given 12 or 6 hourly and in theory should have a more prolonged action than salicylate alone but in practice in most cases there is little to choose between them.

As with all analgesics there is considerable variation in patient preference and one patient will often prefer one preparation when the majority prefer an entirely different one. On several occasions where we have found an analgesic under trial to be ineffective in the majority of patients and have advised against its production and marketing, a few patients have found it helpful and have been disappointed when experimental supplies had to be discontinued.

There is still, therefore, a great need for an effective long-acting non-toxic analgesic preferably with anti-inflammatory properties also, which does not produce gastro-intestinal unwanted effects and is non-addictive. Recurrent and chronic pain is the dominant symptom in almost all the chronic rheumatic disorders, the main recurrent theme in what is often a life-long symphony of suffering. Research into the development and the clinical study of new compounds is still needed as much as it ever was.

REFERENCES

Avioli, L. V. and Berman, M. (1968). *J. Clin. Endocrinol.*, *28*, 700

Barnes, C. G., Turnbull, A. L. and Vernon-Roberts, B. (1971). *Ann. Rheum. Dis.*, *30*, 359

Bell, N. H., Avery, S. and Johnstone, C. (1970). *J. Clin. Endocrinol.*, *31*, 283

Bijvoet, O. L. M. and Jansen, A. P. (1967). *Lancet*, *ii*, 471

Boardman, P. L. and Hart, F. D. (1967). *Brit. Med. J.*, *4*, 265

Charnley, J. (1971). *Ann. Rheum. Dis.*, *30*, 560

Condon, J. R. (1971). *Brit. Med. J.*, *4*, 719

de Haas, W. H. D., de Boer, W., Griffioen, P. and Oosten-Elst, P. (1973). *Ann. Rheum. Dis.*, *32*, 91

Haddad, J. G., Birge, S. J. and Avioli, L. V. (1970). *New Eng. J. Med.*, *283*, 549

Hamrin, B., Jonsson, N. and Landberg, T. (1964). *Lancet*, *i*, 397

Hart, F. D. (1968). *Lancet*, *ii*, 1340

Hart, F. D. (1971). *Clin. Orthopaedics*, *74*, 7

Hart, F. D. (1971). *Brit. Med. J.*, *2*, 210

Hart, F. D. (1973). *French's Index of Differential Diagnosis*. Bristol: John Wright (10th edition), p. 87

Hart, F. D. and Ridgeway, H. J. (1957). *Lancet*, *ii*, 642

Hill, H. (1973). *Lancet*, *i*, 36

Huskisson, E. C. and Hart, F. D. (1972a). *Brit. Med. J.*, *4*, 193

Huskisson, E. C. and Hart, F. D. (1972b). *Ann. Rheum. Dis.*, *31*, 402

Huskisson, E. C. and Hart, F. D. (1973). *Joint Disease: All the Arthropathies*. Bristol: John Wright, in press

Jaffe, I. A. (1970). *Arth. Rheum.*, *13*, 436

Kellgren, J. H. and Moore, R. (1952). *Brit. Med. J.*, *1*, 181

Licht, S. (1968). *Rehabilitation and Medicine*. London: Newhaven (Medical Books) Ltd., p. 15

Scott, W. A. M. (1969). *Practitioner*, *202*, 802

Shearn, M. A. (1972). *Seminars in Arthritis and Rheumatism*, *2*, 165

Sinclair, R. J. G. (1971). *Proc. Roy. Soc. Med.*, *64*, 1031

Wanka, J. and Dixon, A. St. J. (1964). *Ann. Rheum. Dis.*, *23*, 288

Wyke, B. D. (1967). *Ann. Roy. Col. Surg. Eng.*, *41*, 23

Wyke, B. D. (1970). *Rheumatology Phys. Med.*, *10*, 356

4

The Management of Pain in Incurable Malignant Disease

Gerald Westbury

Introduction

The problem of pain in malignant disease is compounded of many factors. Cancers can cause severe pain but many cancers are painless in spite of popular belief to the contrary. It is this popular belief, the expectation that cancer will be painful, that may amplify the patient's awareness of his symptoms. Again, since the diagnosis of cancer is often equated by the sufferer with the prospect of death, fear is a further aggravating factor.

In the management of pain in incurable cancer three main approaches will be discussed.

1. The treatment of the malignant process.
2. The symptomatic management of pain.
3. Terminal care.

It must be emphasized that these divisions, though helpful in the analysis of the problem, are to some extent artificial. Each patient is a complete individual with his own unique physical constitution, family background, pattern of education and religious beliefs. Proper handling of the patient with due concern for all these factors calls for high degrees of medical skill and sympathy.

Treatment of the malignant process

An attempt to provide a comprehensive account of the treatment of neoplasia is neither possible nor desirable within the confines of this text. The practitioner faced with a patient with incurable cancer should however be aware of the range of specific treatment which might have application in the palliation of pain. Such treatment may be surgical, radiotherapeutic or chemotherapeutic.

SURGICAL METHODS

Tumours of the extremities

Amputation of a limb is usually performed with intent to cure but this most irreversible of all operations has a definite place in palliation, even when disease has spread beyond the affected member. Pain, swelling and deformity caused by otherwise uncontrollable primary tumors of bone, soft tissues or skin may call for major ablation and it is remarkable to see how the patient's condition may be transformed thereby. Not only is pain relieved but removal of the useless, sometimes bleeding or infected and generally parasitic limb leads to recovery of general well being with restoration of appetite, weight gain and elevation of hemoglobin level. In spite of the presence of metastases a sufficient length of comfortable life may be provided to justify the fitting of an artificial limb, especially in the young.

Carcinoma of the breast

Cancer within the breast is rarely painful. Locally advanced disease may however cause pain as well as offensive ulceration and discharge and, especially where irradiation has failed, simple mastectomy may afford palliation.

Metastatic breast carcinoma however can cause severe pain, principally when involving the skeleton. The most reliable method of relief is irradiation of the painful site but this is not feasible where disease is widespread because of the risk of generalized bone marrow damage. Removal of the ovaries in pre-menopausal women, or the adrenals in older women, or removal or destruction of the pituitary gland, may produce immediate relief of pain with healing of all lesions in about 30% of cases. The period of remission is variable but in a small number of patients can last up to ten years or more.

Carcinoma of the prostate

Like the breast, carcinoma of the prostate is a hormone dependent tumor and bilateral orchidectomy is often dramatically effective in relieving the pain of skeletal metastases, as well as reducing the bulk of the primary tumor and so contributing to the control of urinary symptoms. The value of bilateral adrenalectomy or hypophysectomy when orchidectomy (or hormones) are no longer effective is less certain than in the case of breast cancer.

Gastrointestinal cancer

The palliative surgery of this group of diseases is mainly concerned with the relief of obstruction, which in itself is a source of pain. Nowhere is the value of this type of surgery better seen than in advanced rectal cancer where tenesmus and diarrhea reduce the patient to a state of misery. A simple relieving colostomy diverts the fecal stream with reduction of sepsis and edema around the tumor, and consequent amelioration of symptoms. Even when the rectum is irremovable, colostomy seems sometimes to slow down the rate of growth and may allow months or years of comfortable life. For low rectal carcinomas, additional diathermy coagulation may extend the period of comfortable control.

Carcinoma of the lung

The place of surgery for the relief of pain is confined to treatment of the peripheral carcinoma which has invaded the chest wall. Resection of the affected lung or lobe in continuity with the invaded parietes is indicated, and may result in long survival or cure. Unfortunately the Pancoast or upper pulmonary sulcus tumor, which causes severe pain by invasion of the brachial plexus, is not amenable to surgical attack.

Carcinoma of the tongue, mouth and jaws

Palliative surgery is to be considered when radiotherapy has failed to relieve pain. Operation may occasionally take the form of formal resection but is more likely to entail less formidable procedures such as local excision, diathermy coagulation, the removal of sequestrated bone or drainage, e.g. as in palatal fenestration of the maxillary antrum.

It is particularly in this region that the technique of cryosurgery has proved of value for the palliation of inoperable malignant disease. The tumor is frozen in a controlled manner using a partially insulated probe whose tip is cooled by circulation of liquid nitrogen to a temperature of $-195.8\,°C$. Destruction by freezing carries several advantages, including anesthesia of the 'cryolesion' during and after the procedure, and absence of bleeding.

RADIOTHERAPY

Ionizing radiation is used in the relief of pain due to malignant disease because of its preferential biological effect in destroying malignant cells. Radiation for palliation is usually delivered by external beam either from an x-ray machine or a radioactive source, e.g. the cobalt-60 bomb. Less often small radioactive sources in the form of 'seeds' or 'needles' can be implanted directly into the tumor.

Among the more radiosensitive of primary tumors may be listed the lymphomas and reticuloses, seminoma of the testis and myeloma. Intermediate in radiosensitivity follow carcinomas of the skin and epidermoid carcinomas of the mucous membranes, carcinomas of the cervix and bladder and some carcinomas of the lung and breast. At the most radio-resistant end of the scale are some adenocarcinomas of the gastrointestinal system, sarcomas of bone and soft tissue and most malignant melanomas.

The pain of localized metastatic deposits in bone most commonly originating from primary tumors in the breast and lung is readily and regularly controlled by radiation. This perhaps is the most rewarding field of pain relief in cancer treated by the radiotherapist.

Severe headache from intracranial metastases often yields to external irradiation, though temporary loss of hair is an unpleasant sequel.

In breast cancer, irradiation of the ovaries to an adequate dose is as effective as surgical castration, but the results in terms of reduction of hormone production and consequent palliation are not fully effective for at least six weeks.

Modern radiotherapeutic techniques have reduced some of the unpleasant side effects of treatment. Supervoltage x-rays, that is x-rays generated at more than 1 million volts, and the comparable gamma emissions of, e.g. cobalt-60 sources cause much less skin reaction than do 'conventional' x-ray beams. These higher energy rays are also less damaging to bone, a property of great value when treating, for instance carcinoma of the lower alveolus invading the mandible.

According to orthodox practice, radiation was delivered in relatively small daily fractions over several weeks. It is now appreciated that equivalent effects can be produced by fewer, larger fractions given at longer intervals. This reduction in the number and frequency of treatments has obvious advantages for the out-patient being managed from his home.

CHEMOTHERAPY
Under this heading will be considered the use of hormones and of cytotoxic agents.

HORMONAL THERAPY

Carcinoma of the breast
This is the best known example of a malignant tumor which can be influenced by hormonal manipulation, whether by removal or destruction of endocrine glands (*vide supra*) or by administration of hormones or hormone blocking agents. Roughly 30 to 40% of breast cancers are hormone dependent. The problem is to know which patient will respond, and in that case, which is the hormonal method of choice. Rapidly evolving disease, as when the interval between treatment of the primary and the appearance of metastases is less than a year, is less likely to respond than disease recurring after many years free interval. Breast cancer in the first 5 years following the menopause is also usually refractory to hormonal manipulation.

As a general rule androgens, or preferably their non-masculinizing derivatives are recommended before the menopause and estrogens after, but in practice this rule does not always apply. Occasionally androgens or estrogens may provoke disease and this is an indication for changing to an alternative hormone. The risk of provocation calls for careful observation at the outset of treatment, not only for obvious exacerbation of soft tissue deposits or increase in bone pain, but because rapid elevation in serum calcium level may produce severe systemic disturbance and renal failure.

In addition to androgens and estrogens, cortisone and its analogues and progestogens may be effective. More recently agents have been introduced which block the peripheral action of estrogens.

To a large extent the selection of hormone or hormonal surgical procedure has been a question of rule of thumb. Measurement of the ratio of androgen:corticosteroid metabolites in the patient's urine is of some predictive value for the outcome of hormonal manipulation, but this does not really help in the management of the individual case. Recent work on the *in vitro* response to various hormones of breast cancer biopsy specimens has raised hopes that it will be possible not only to foretell which patients will respond, but in addition to know which particular treatment is best suited to the individual patient.

Carcinoma of the prostate
This was the first cancer to be treated by hormones, and approximately 80% of patients respond favorably either to estrogens or to castration. Response is shown by reduction and disappearance of bone pain, regression of the primary tumor and fall in serum acid phosphatase level, which can be a useful monitor of progress. Estrogens may produce untoward side effects such as painful enlargement of the breasts and, more seriously, sodium and water retention which can precipitate congestive cardiac failure in this generally elderly group of patients. The presence of cardiac decompensation is the most important indication for surgical castration in preference to the administration of estrogens.

Other cancers
Certain other malignant tumors may respond to endocrine therapy, though with less certainty than the prostate or breast. They include carcinomas of the endometrium, kidney and thyroid, and teratoma of the testis. The leukemias and reticuloses can be favorably influenced by corticosteroid therapy and these agents are commonly incorporated in the multiple drug schedules now in use.

CYTOTOXIC THERAPY
This form of treatment for cancer originated from experiments on mustard gas derivatives in the Second World War, producing the prototype cytotoxic agent, nitrogen mustard. Since that time many thousands of compounds with anti-cancer

properties have been elaborated and several dozens of these are in current use.

Classification

Cytotoxic drugs fall into five main groups:

1. Alkylating agents. These include the nitrogen mustards (e.g. mustine, chlorambucil, melphalan, cyclophosphamide), thiotepa, busulphan and ethoglucid. They act directly on the chemical constituents of the malignant cell, especially DNA. Their common mode of action and hence their generic name is the replacement of a hydrogen atom in the target molecule by an alkyl radical.

2. Antimetabolites. These are synthetic compounds designed to mimic essential normal cell constituents so closely that they 'fraudulently' take over the enzymes concerned with nucleic acid synthesis. This process of competition thus blocks the normal metabolic pathway for production of DNA, and is especially damaging to rapidly dividing cells. They include folic acid antagonists (e.g. methotrexate), purine antagonists (e.g. mercaptopurine) and the pyrimidine antagonists (e.g. fluorouracil).

3. Plant alkaloids. These include certain colchicine derivatives and the Vinca alkaloids, vinblastine and vincristine. They act on cell nuclei in mitosis blocking division during metaphase.

4. Antibiotics. These are substances derived from micro-organisms and include the actinomycosins C and D, daunorubicin, mithramycin, mitomycin and streptozotocin. Their modes of action on cell division are complex and incompletely understood.

5. Miscellaneous. Here are included some relatively simple low molecular weight compounds, e.g. urethane, hydroxyurea and procarbazine.

Use of cytotoxic drugs

This is a complex matter and must be managed and often administered by specialized hospital staff. For this reason details of choice of agent and dosage will not be given, but rather general principles outlined.

Agents may be used singly but selected combinations of two, three or more, usually of different class, can enhance therapeutic effect without increasing toxicity. Therapy may be given continuously, or in intermittent intensive 'pulsed' courses with rest periods in between.

Drugs such as mustine, the Vinca alkaloids and the actinomycosins can only be administered by the intravenous route. Chlorambucil is given by mouth. Melphalan, cyclophosphamide and methotrexate may be given orally or intravenously.

Though best known in the treatment of the leukemias and lymphomas, it is now appreciated that these agents, especially used in combination, can produce substantial alleviation of symptoms in some carcinomas and less often in some sarcomas. Thus, for example, more than 75% of advanced breast cancers respond usefully to a four drug regime (methotrexate, vincristine, cyclophosphamide, fluorouracil) given as a 5-day course each month. Cytotoxic therapy is also useful, though less consistently than in the case of the breast for palliation of cancer of the lung, gastrointestinal tract, ovary and testicle, and in Wilm's tumor, Ewing's tumor and certain other sarcomas of childhood.

The effect of cytotoxic agents is seen especially on rapidly dividing cells and as would be expected toxicity is expressed mainly in the bone marrow, gastrointestinal lining epithelium and hair follicles. Toxic side effects vary from drug to drug and patients show variation in response, some withstanding intensive therapy with little complaint. However malaise, nausea and vomiting, diarrhea, ulceration of the mouth, and loss of hair can cause distress. The blood count must be monitored regularly during treatment with special reference to the level of circulating white cells and platelets.

The initiation of cytotoxic therapy is sometimes best conducted in hospital, but with good collaboration between specialist, general practitioner and the pathology laboratory maintenance can be continued on an out-patient basis. In this respect the use of orally administered drugs, where appropriate, is clearly advantageous.

Regional intra-arterial cytotoxic therapy
This embraces a variety of methods by which cytotoxic agents in high concentration are introduced directly into the artery

supplying a tumor bearing region with consequent reduction of systemic toxicity.

The technique of isolated extracorporeal perfusion involves surgical cannulation of the main artery and vein, and artificial maintenance for an hour or so of the part thus supplied, by means of a pump-oxygenator. In the case of the limbs, this now independently perfused region can be effectively isolated from the general circulation by a proximally placed tourniquet, and high doses of cytotoxic agent infused with minimal overspill to the rest of the patient. Isolated perfusion with melphalan is a valuable means of control of locally advanced malignant melanoma of the limbs.

The simpler intra-arterial injection or infusion is effected by introducing a fine plastic cannula into the appropriate artery, either by open operation or preferably, and where possible, by percutaneous puncture. Drugs are injected intermittently or infused continuously using a pump. Intra-arterial infusion may be of palliative value in advanced cancers of the face, mouth and jaws (external carotid artery) and in liver cancer both primary and secondary (hepatic artery). Although usually a hospital procedure, infusion can be conducted on ambulant out-patients over many months using portable miniaturized pumps. The pain of advanced cancer of the pelvic viscera is often temporarily eased by intermittent injection of, e.g. mustine, into the lower abdominal aorta through a catheter introduced via simple puncture of the femoral artery in the groin. Inflation of thigh tourniquets above arterial pressure during the period of the injection helps limit distribution of the drug mainly to the pelvis.

Symptomatic management of pain

The symptomatic management of malignant disease is influenced greatly by the limited prognosis of the sufferer. This is true for the pharmacological aspect, where the implications of drug dependence are much less important than in patients with normal life expectancy and pain of non-malignant origin. It is also true with regard to selection of the various pain pathway interruption procedures available. In patients with advanced cancer minor procedures are preferable to major surgical interventions and measures which bring adequate relief for short periods, e.g. only weeks or months may yet be appropriate.

It must be recognized, however, that some advanced malignancies do run a long course and the prescription must be tempered to the individual requirement.

INTERRUPTION OF PAIN CONDUCTING PATHWAYS

This approach is considered first, not because it is more important or necessarily preferable, but in order to emphasize that where indicated it should be applied early before the patient's spirit and endurance have been broken by long periods of useless suffering. Indeed the results of these procedures are often disappointing when used as a last resort.

The scope and technique of the methods available are discussed in detail in Chapters 5 and 6. In summary the sensory pathways may be interrupted at the level of the peripheral nerves, distally or in their short course within the spinal canal; at the level of the ascending spinal tracts; and within the brainstem and the brain itself. The procedure itself may be non-surgical (peripheral nerve and plexus blocks; intrathecal blocks, intrathecal osmotic neurolysis and barbotage) or surgical (nerve section; ganglionectomy; posterior rhizotomy; cordotomy; brainstem tractotomy; open surgical or stereotactic interruption of intracerebral pathways from the level of the basal ganglia to the sensory cortex). For obvious reasons non-operative or minor surgical measures are usually to be preferred in patients with incurable cancer.

The nerves of the head and neck and the intercostal nerves are accessible for peripheral block or section. The pain to be treated must be reasonably well localized and it is usual to precede the definitive procedure by a trial block with local anesthetic.

Coeliac plexus block by paravertebral injection of neurolytic agents such as phenol may help the pain of inoperable carcinoma of the stomach or pancreas, but it will relieve pain only of visceral origin, pain due to infiltration of the posterior parietes remaining unaffected.

Intrathecal injection of neurolytic agents, e.g. phenol in glycerine or alcohol is a simple technique, though accurate placing by positioning of the patient is essential. The period of relief obtained is variable and spread of the solution to motor elements may cause weakness or paralysis of the limbs or bladder.

Intrathecal injection of ice cold or hypertonic saline may also give useful though variable pain relief for weeks or a few months and, like the injection of neurolytic solutions, can easily be repeated when the effect wears off. General anesthesia is required. Barbotage, or the simple withdrawal and replacement of cerebro-spinal fluid through a wide bore needle has been recently claimed to produce similar effects, and has the advantage that no special apparatus is required and furthermore general anesthesia is unnecessary. The mode of action of this and of hyperosmotic therapy is not fully understood.

Posterior spinal rhizotomy is sometimes indicated for the pain of malignant disease confined to a localized segment of the body, especially for segmental pain affecting the chest or abdominal wall. At least five roots must be divided for effective relief because of the overlap between adjacent dermatomes. The operation involves exposure of the spinal cord by laminectomy and division of the relevant dorsal roots after their careful separation from the corresponding motor roots. Rhizotomy is applicable wherever the component roots can be identified. Sensory rhizotomy of the fifth and ninth cranial nerves, together with the second, third and fourth cervical nerves, may be used for severe pain in the jaw and neck. Rhizotomy in the dorsal or lumbar regions will be selected for pain of appropriate root distribution. Division of the second, third and fourth sacral roots together with interruption of the hypogastric plexus may be used for the alleviation of severe pelvic pain, e.g. inoperable cancer of uterus or bladder.

Cordotomy selectively interrupts pain (and temperature) pathways in the opposite half of the body from a few segments below the level of section. The surgical operation is performed in the cervical region for pain in the arm and upper trunk and in the dorsal region for pain affecting the lower back, abdomen or pelvis. Bilateral cervical cordotomy may cause trouble by temporary interference with respiratory movements, as may even unilateral cordotomy if disease has already reduced pulmonary function. Bilateral cordotomy at any level can lead to retention of urine and severe constipation which may be permanent in up to 10% of patients. The more recently evolved technique of percutaneous cervical cordotomy has the advantages of avoidance of open operation and general anesthesia. In good hands the efficacy and risks are comparable to those of open surgery and furthermore the pain of laminectomy is avoided. This technique therefore represents an obvious advance, especially in patients with mortal disease.

Pain control by destruction of higher centers is seldom applicable to patients with malignant disease and certainly procedures such as leukotomies with their tendency to produce depersonalization will be used with the utmost reluctance. It has been rightly said that palliative surgery for pain is not a substitute for the general understanding of the patient and his problems.

TREATMENT BY DRUGS

It must be made clear at outset that the treatment of pain by drugs cannot be dissociated from the general management of the patient and his problems. Pain is a complex function whose physical and psychological elements are not readily separated. Chronic pain produces depression and distress and itself is increased by fear and isolation. Realization by the patient that he has cancer is associated with fear of death and fear that this death will be a painful one. The response of the patient to pain relieving medication depends greatly on the attitude of the prescriber — the value of the placebo cannot be underestimated. No one has contributed more to the subject of control of pain and distress in late malignant disease than Dr Cicely Saunders, whose teaching has greatly influenced those aspects dealt with in this chapter. The key to success in medication is constant control of pain. Prescription strictly by the clock has no place in this scheme. Analgesics must be given frequently enough to be effective before pain recurs. The oral route of administration is obviously preferable and is usually adequate provided pain is not allowed to get out of hand. When the patient has confidence that he will not be left to suffer until some appointed hour for his next dose, the vicious circle of anxiety—pain—misery can be broken, and relief achieved often by surprisingly small amounts of drug.

The entire pharmacopeia is at the disposal of the doctor treating pain. Patients vary greatly in the potency of analgesia required and this together with the dosage necessary also vary from time to time in the same person. Again individual analgesics may have different effects in different patients. Rather than exploring the broad range of medication available, the practitioner is well advised to select a few useful analgesics and to become thoroughly conversant with their use and side effects.

The effect of analgesic agents is augmented by various drugs which act on mood. Such adjuvants are very valuable in increasing the efficacy and reducing the dose of analgesics but are no substitute for exercise of patience and understanding on the part of the doctor and nurse.

Analgesics
The control of pain in cancer does not always require the use of the more powerful narcotic analgesics. Among the group of mild analgesics aspirin in soluble form, alone or in combination, is valuable, though the possibility of gastric irritation must be borne in mind. Paracetamol 500 mg (Panadol) is useful and may be combined with dextropropoxyphene (Doloxene) as Distalgesic.

Analgesics of intermediate strength include pentazocine (Fortral) 25–100 mg by mouth or 30–60 mg i.m. injection, dihydrocodeine (DF118) 30–60 mg orally or 20–50 mg i.m. and dextromoramide (Palfium) 5–10 mg by mouth.

Where powerful analgesia is called for, pethidine (Demerol) 50–200 mg by mouth or 50–150 mg i.m. or methadone (Physeptone) 5–10 mg orally can be useful, but morphine, initially 10 mg and diamorphine (heroin) initially 5–10 mg by mouth or 3–6 mg s.c. will often be necessary. With these drugs the central analgesic affect is enhanced by the sedation and sense of mental detachment also produced. Morphine has the disadvantages of erratic absorption by the oral route and a tendency to produce nausea and constipation. Heroin is preferable in all these respects and also causes less mental clouding. Its reputedly greater addictive property is seldom a disadvantage in the type of patient under discussion. Morphine and heroin are used in the various recipes for the 'Brompton

Cocktail'. They are potentiated by the phenothiazine group of drugs, e.g. chlorpromazine, which in addition lessen their tendency to produce nausea and vomiting.

Drugs influencing mood

Anxiety, tension and agitation magnify the impact of pain; tranquillizers and anxiolytic drugs therefore have a place in combination with analgesics in its management. Chlorpromazine (Largactil) initially 25 mg orally, i.m. or i.v. is the most widely used member of the phenothiazine group. Its value in combination with morphine has already been described and it is especially suited to the elderly agitated patient. Perphenazine (Fentazin) 4–8 mg; prochlorperazine (Stemetil) 10–30 mg; and trifluoperazine (Stelazine) 1–6 mg have more potent anti-emetic effect but like all the phenothiazines may produce depression or Parkinsonism. Among the benzodiazepine group are included chlordiazepoxide (Librium) 10–100 mg daily; diazepam (Valium) 5–30 mg daily and nitrazepam (Mogadon) 5–10 mg. Nitrazepam is a most valuable hypnotic and in this respect the importance of sleep cannot be too strongly emphasized.

Where pain is associated with depression, the tricyclic antidepressants have their place along with the analgesics. Imipramine (Tofranil) 75–150 mg daily and amitryptyline (Tryptizol) 50–150 mg daily are in common use. These drugs may produce drowsiness, blurring of vision, constipation and dizziness.

In this context mention must also be made of alcohol which is an invaluable hypnotic, as well as a constituent of the various forms of Brompton mixture.

With the aid of adjuvant drugs as indicated, and given regularly as required, surprisingly small doses of analgesics may suffice, and even if morphine or heroin are needed, and it is relatively uncommon to require high doses, drug dependence is seldom a problem. This is certainly the case for the short period of life remaining to most patients with disseminated neoplasia.

After all that has been written on the pharmacology of pain, the importance of the conviction of the prescribing doctor must again be stressed. It has been rightly said that the physician must give a little of himself along with every prescription.

The management of distress in the terminal phase

Discussion of these aspects under a separate heading is artificial because they are inseparable from the foregoing. Pain itself and often the knowledge by the sufferer that he has cancer are distressing at all stages, but the approach of death introduces special considerations.

Quite simple mechanical problems can contribute to the overall picture of misery and are equally simply relieved if looked for. Constipation, pressure sores, unpleasant discharges and odors all yield to skilled nursing. An indwelling catheter may ease the burden of repeated calls for bedpan or bottle. These measures along with intelligent control of pain help to bolster the dignity of the individual.

Nausea is a more troublesome complaint though modern anti-emetic drugs are helpful. Dyspnea is one of the most distressing of all symptoms and, if pleural effusion is contributary, tapping will be gratefully welcomed. Where such direct help is not applicable, morphine in sedative dosage should not be withheld.

More than anything the patient is in need of human contact and understanding from doctors and nurses who are prepared to visit him regularly and allow the necessary time to listen. There is a great temptation on the part of the medical attendant to avoid the dying patient. This reluctance in confrontation arises partly because death is unpleasant and partly because the very situation of the patient implies that the medical team has failed. The hospital consultant is perhaps especially guilty in this respect and all too often fails to appreciate, for instance, the impact of a whispered conversation with the junior and nursing staff at the foot of the bed with barely a glance at the patient. Patients look forward to the regular medical round and prefer to be woken if asleep, rather than passed by. Failure to observe these considerations gives rise to the impression in the patient's mind that his case is a hopeless one, and the sense of isolation thereby engendered can never be counter-balanced by any amount of skilled pharmacology.

Where should patients be cared for in this final stage of

their illness? There are strong arguments in favor of the home, not the least being the services and very presence of the family practitioner. Nursing requirements however may make home care difficult and bearing in mind too the great stress placed on the family, hospitalization may be required. The type of hospital available depends on the local district resources. Sadly the acute general hospital is, for reasons mentioned, not always the best fitted for this function and there is much to be said for the purpose built home, of which St Christopher's Hospice, Sydenham, London, is such a fine example. In such institutions the benefits of specialized knowledge in the management of terminal cases is seen in the remarkable change brought about in those hopeless and pain ridden sufferers admitted to their care. Indeed the combination of cheerful confidence, skill in the management of physical symptoms, and devotion of time to what may be termed problems of the spirit may enable patients to return to their homes for worthwhile periods of time. The knowledge that they can come back to the institution if the situation were to prove too much to bear is often sufficient to sustain them contentedly in the family environment.

RECOMMENDED READING

Ackerman, L. V. and del Regato, J. A. (1970). *Cancer. Diagnosis, Treatment and Prognosis.* St. Louis: The C. V. Mosby Co.

Boesen, E. and Davis, W. (1969). *Cytotoxic Drugs in the Treatment of Cancer.* London: Edward Arnold

Laurence, D. R. (1973). *Clinical Pharmacology.* Edinburgh: Churchill Livingstone

Saunders, C. (1966). The Management of Terminal Illness. *Hospital Medicine, 1,* 225, 317, 443

Stoll, B. A. (editor) (1972). *Endocrine Therapy in Malignant Disease.* Philadelphia: W. B. Saunders Co. Ltd.

5

Neurosurgical Treatment of Pain in Neuralgias of Non-Malignant Etiology

James C. White

Introduction

Pain of the type discussed in this chapter rarely subsides spontaneously. It is often so severe that the victim becomes totally incapacitated and frequently addicted to narcotics. Mental depression is often an added factor. Nine of the victims whom we have been unable to relieve have committed suicide. The possibility of surgical relief should therefore be considered at an early stage. Prior to referring these sufferers to a neurosurgeon it is often advisable to obtain the advice of an experienced psychiatrist to decide whether the patient is exaggerating his symptoms in order to obtain his accustomed medication. The general practitioner should also realize that pain may be purely psychogenic. When a psychosomatic background has been ruled out, a gratifying number of sufferers can be relieved by surgery and will promptly stop their demands for analgesic drugs.

At the Massachusetts General Hospital we have operated on over a thousand such patients with satisfactory outcome in 74%. The most common causes for their distress were peripheral nerve or sensory root scarring resulting from trauma, previous surgery or disease. Central pain due to cerebral or spinal lesions was another, less frequent cause. In a considerable number, however, the etiological factor was unknown. This applies particularly to the cases of trigeminal and other cephalic neuralgias. My experience with relief of pain has been reviewed in a recent monograph with Sweet (White and Sweet, 1969). We have followed most of our patients over a period of years. This is the only way of telling whether neurosurgical treatment is effective. The great majority of carefully selected subjects were relieved at first, but in approximately one quarter

113

pain eventually recurred. The reason for this is that in patients with a normal life-expectancy nature has a remarkable capacity of developing new pathways for the conduction of pain; also after axons are cut distal to their sensory root ganglia regeneration may take place.

It has been our policy to discuss the problems related to surgical relief with every patient in detail, telling each the chances of lasting success and possible failure; also the risks of major complications. The patient alone knows the exact intensity of his suffering and is in a position to decide whether he wishes to take the necessary gamble of obtaining freedom from his pain. We recommend major surgical intervention only when the pain is obviously intolerable or the patient is threatened with addiction or severe depression.

Owing to limitation of space it is not feasible to include some of the rarer causes of chronic pain. It is also not possible to give a detailed description of surgical technique, but in order to give the general practitioner some idea of the operations mentioned below, their extent, complications and general effectiveness, a brief summary is included at the end of this chapter. For a more detailed description the interested reader should refer to the monograph on pain by White and Sweet (1969), or to the recent volume on neurosurgery edited by Youmans (1973).

The cephalic neuralgias (Table 5.1)

TRIGEMINAL NEURALGIA (*TIC DOULOUREUX*)

Clinical description

Tic douloureux, as its name implies, consists of sudden, severe stabs of pain in one or more divisions of the trigeminal nerve. This neuralgia usually starts in the latter half of life and is characteristically triggered by tactile or postural stimuli, on touching the skin, shaving, brushing the teeth, or on eating or talking. In the rare cases of bilateral tic (3%) the flashes of pain occur on only one side of the face at a time.

The distribution of pain is usually limited to one or two divisions of the nerve, mandibular and maxillary or supra-orbital and maxillary. It rarely involves all three branches of the trigeminus.

There is no neurological deficit. When the pain is continuous, gives rise to cutaneous or corneal numbness or dysesthesia, or spreads beyond the trigeminal area, one must search for some other diagnosis.

Surgical treatment

1. *Peripheral procedures*—Peripheral nerve block has long been carried out by injecting alcohol at the supraorbital notch and into the infraorbital foramen, or more centrally where the mandibular division emerges from the skull at the foramen ovale. The maxillary division can be similarly blocked in the pterygomaxillary fossa. Stabs of pain can also be stopped by

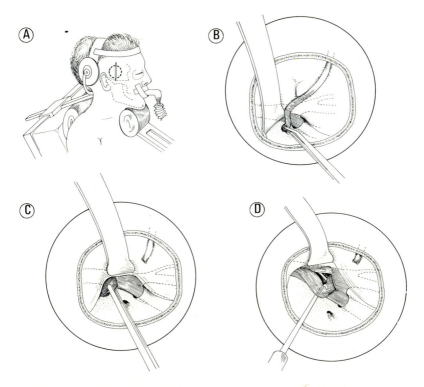

Figure 5.1   Retrogasserian rhizotomy. A. Position of patient. B. Plugging foramen spinosum prior to coagulation and section of middle meningeal artery. C. Separation of temporal lobe dura from ganglion and root sheath. D. Separation of 2nd and 3rd division fibers with preservation of 1st division and underlying motor root.

Table 5.1 RESULTS OF SURGICAL TREATMENT OF TRIGEMINAL NEURALGIA

These statistics are based on Dr W. H. Sweet's review of case reports from leading neurosurgical clinics in England, Europe and North America

Method	No. of cases	Mortality	Early relief	Recurrence	Paresthesia, mild	Anesthesia dolorosa	Facial paralysis, permanent	Keratitis	Paralysis of other cranial nerves	Miscellaneous complications
Subtemporal rhizotomy (Frazier)	5,439	2%	95%	15%	15%	3%	3%	5%	1%	
Suboccipital rhizotomy (Dandy)	716	4%	100%	25%	20%	2.4%	2%	5%	0	
Compression or decompression of sensory root (Shelden et al.) (Pudenz and Shelden)	811	1%	97%	23%	rare	very rare	2%	0	rare	
Descending Vth tractomy (Sjöqvist)	926	1.6%	89%	13%	25%	0.5%	0	0.1%	rare hoarseness	lateropulsion and unsteady gait 9%, brachial ataxia 6%

Table 5.1 (continued)

Method	No. of cases	Mortality	Early relief	Recurrence	Paresthesia, mild	Anesthesia dolorosa	Facial paralysis, permanent	Keratitis	Paralysis of other cranial nerves	Miscellaneous complications
Alcohol injection of sensory root (Harris)	367	0	—	14%	'small proportion'	—	—	—	—	no statistics on complications
(Penman)	100	0	97%	15%	—	—	0	15%	2%	
Phenol injection of sensory root (Jefferson)	50	0	98%	28%	—	0	0	0	0	
Electrocoagulation of sensory root (Thiry)	100	0	100%	29%*	20%	0	0	0	0?	
Heating sensory root by radio-frequency current (Sweet and Wepsic)	274	0	94%	22%	—	0	0	0.4%	0	loss of corneal reflex 5%, only one corneal ulceration

* All recurrences relieved by recoagulation

cutting the supra- or infraorbital nerve; also by cutting the inferior alveolar and lingual branches when the lower lip, jaw and tongue are involved. While no peripheral procedures are likely to give relief for more than a year or two at the most, they are often useful to show the patient what permanent numbness that follows rhizotomy will be like and also to give an exhausted elderly patient a reprieve.

2. *Retrogasserian rhizotomy* — In order to prevent regeneration of the peripheral portion of a nerve its central fibers must be interrupted proximally to the sensory root ganglion. For many years the standard operation was Frazier's (1925) retrogasserian rhizotomy by the subtemporal approach (see Figure 5.1). In skilled hands partial section permits sparing the first division fibers with the corneal reflex as well as the motor root. Recent modifications which are safer and carry less hazards of complications are now making this procedure obsolete. Results of retrogasserian rhizotomy together with postoperative complications are summarized in Table 5.1. These statistics are taken from Dr Sweet's review of 5,439 cases which have been reported by leading neurosurgeons over the past 35 years (White and Sweet, 1969). They include our experience with 605 patients. It will be seen that early relief is nearly always obtained, but that up to 15% have an eventual return of attacks. This can occur when the sensory fibers are cut too close to the ganglion, permitting a few ganglion cells to remain attached to their central processes. In these circumstances the peripheral end of the neurone can regenerate. Operative mortality has amounted to less than 2%. The chief complications are annoying 'crawling' paresthesiae in some 15% to more serious anesthesia dolorosa, and paralytic keratitis in approximately 5%. Other rare but serious complications are hemiplegia, aphasia and injury to other cranial nerves. Facial paralysis has occurred in 3%, but has been permanent in only 1%. Injury to branches of the nerves to the extraocular muscles, which lie just medial to the ganglion within the cavernous sinus, has been reported in 1%.

The sensory root can also be cut by a suboccipital route as it enters the brain stem in the upper pons (see Figure 5.2). This approach is more difficult. It carries twice the risk of mortality and is no more free of complications. Furthermore, it does not permit a selective section of the root fibers. It has only two advantages: the motor root, which leaves the pons at

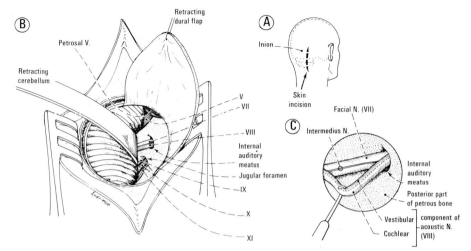

Figure 5.2 Suboccipital exposure of pain-conducting cranial nerves.
A. Position of incision. B. Anatomical relations of cranial nerves V, VII, VIII, IX, X
and XI. C. Relation of nervus intermedius to facial and acoustic nerves.

a slightly higher level, is never paralyzed; and it occasionally
discloses an aneurysm or tumor compressing the nerve beneath
the tentorium.

In the 3% of individuals with neuralgia involving both
sides of the face, bilateral rhizotomy must be avoided. With loss
of position sense on both sides the individual is unaware of the
location of food in his mouth or whether saliva is drooling from
his lips.

3. *Other operations for permanently interrupting the posterior root
fibers* — Numerous other techniques have been devised and
given extended trial to simplify and safeguard the relief of
trigeminal neuralgia. The most urgent needs are to protect the
patient against paralysis of other cranial nerves, paralytic
keratitis with possible loss of vision, and the extremely disagreeable paresthesias that may follow numbness of the face.
Space does not permit a detailed description of each method,
but the overall results are summarized in Table 5.1.

Decompression or compression of the root fibers, advocated
by Pudenz and Shelden (1952) and Shelden (1966): These
operations consist of lysis of the ganglion and its root fibers in
Meckel's cave and/or gentle compression. They do not produce
total anesthesia and thus nearly obviate the risk of keratitis
and severe paresthesia, but they are followed by a relatively
high incidence of recurrence.

Tractotomy of the descending bulbo-spinal sensory tract (Sjöqvist, 1949) is discussed below under glossopharyngeal-vagal neuralgia. Its advantages are that it does not take away sense of touch or position and it is rarely followed by paresthesia or keratitis. There is also no risk of paralyzing the muscles of mastication. Although the mortality rate is low, the operation takes a great deal out of the patient and it is occasionally followed by ataxia of the arm and lateral deviation of gait. Its only justification at present is in the rare (3%) cases of bilateral neuralgia, when it is so important that the patient retain sense of touch and position on at least one side of the tongue and jaw.

4. *Injection procedures* — Injection of alcohol by inserting the needle through the foramen ovale into the Gasserian ganglion and its root fibers in Meckel's cave is a potentially dangerous procedure. In the reports of experts such as Harris (1940) and Penman (1953) the results were nearly as good as those after rhizotomy. There were no deaths and no greater incidence of serious complications. However, in less expert hands the risks of spilling alcohol out of the root sleeve and paralyzing other cranial nerves were prohibitive. These hazards can be reduced, but not altogether eliminated, by Jaeger's (1959) use of boiling water. If injection by neurotoxic solutions is desirable, Jefferson's (1966) use of 5% phenol in glycerine seems most logical. This solution is less diffusible than alcohol and, being heavier than cerebrospinal fluid, can be more readily trapped in the root sheath by gravity. The reported results are impressive with only a 2% rate of failure and no corneal ulceration or anesthesia dolorosa. An added advantage of phenol is that there is usually some preservation of facial sensation, as there is some dissociation between the loss of touch and pain. Only 24% of his subjects had real numbness in two or three divisions and a reduction in the corneal reflex.

5. *Electrocoagulation of the ganglion* — The technique of coagulation of the sensory root fibers has now been so improved that its results are better than those of surgical rhizotomy. With Thiry's method (Thiry, 1962) of inserting the needle electrode through the foramen ovale into the root sheath and gradual heating, all of his first 100 patients have had lasting relief after

one or more coagulations without any serious complications. As sensory loss in his subjects has been carried only to a mild hypesthesia, paresthesia has not been a serious complaint and anesthesia dolorosa has been eliminated. These results have been so good that other forms of surgical treatment have been abandoned in his clinic.

The same is true on our service at the Massachusetts General Hospital, with Dr Sweet's further improvement of controlled radiofrequency coagulation of the desired portion of the sensory root (White and Sweet, 1969; Sweet and Wepsic, 1974). This consists of inserting a needle electrode with a thermister tip and heating to 50–100 °C in stages. With the intermittent use of short-acting intravenous anesthesia (Brevital, methohexital) it is possible to awaken the patient for testing at repeated intervals. The needle insertion is controlled radiographically (Figure 5.3). This places it within the root sleeve where it can be manipulated into the desired portion of the sensory fibers and its position checked by electrical stimulation.

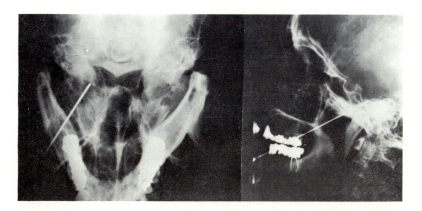

Figure 5.3   Insertion of needle through foramen ovale into trigeminal root sheath under radiographic control. Left: Basal projection showing needle passing through foramen ovale. Right: Lateral view with needle advanced 5 mm beyond profile of clivus almost to porus trigemini. Coagulation at this point caused sensory loss in V_1 and V_2. Needle should be withdrawn so that tip lies anterior to profile of clivus for injection or for coagulation of V_2 and V_3 divisions.

From Sweet and Wepsic, *Journal of Neurosurgery*, in press, by kind permission of the editor.

By heating for successive periods of $\frac{1}{2}$ to 1 minute and awakening the patient for testing the extent and degree of sensory loss, it is usually possible to obtain relief of pain in the desired divisions without producing total anesthesia. Awareness of touch and position sense can usually be preserved as the larger myelinated axons are more resistant to heating. In their first 274 patients lasting relief has been achieved at the first trial in 94%, half of whom have been followed for $2\frac{1}{2}$ to 6 years. There were 22% of late recurrences requiring further treatment. In the 6% of initial failures it has been possible to obtain relief by subsequent coagulation. This procedure requires only overnight hospitalization. It has led to no extra-trigeminal complications. The motor root is usually preserved and there has been only a single instance of corneal ulceration. Also, there have been no complaints of severe paresthesia.

GLOSSOPHARYNGEAL-VAGAL NEURALGIA

Clinical description
This syndrome of intense bursts of pain in the throat has many of the characteristics of *tic douloureux*, with which it is occasionally associated. It is triggered by swallowing and contact or taste of food. Yawning or sneezing may set off an attack. The pain is felt from the back of the tongue, tonsillar fossa, and posterior pharyngeal wall down as far as the larynx. Occasionally it is referred to the aural canal and skin around its orifice. A rare and bizarre variation of these attacks is episodes of cardiac arrest with syncope and sometimes convulsions. These are caused by spread of action potentials to the carotid sinus nerve of Hering and resultant vagal asystole.

Surgical treatment
Formerly it was believed that this form of neuralgia was purely of glossopharyngeal origin, but in order to obtain satisfactory results the surgeon must also interrupt the sensory upper rootlets of the vagus whenever their stimulation in the awakened patient evokes his pain. Interruption of the pain fibers can be carried out in two ways:
    1. By cutting the sensory root of the glossopharyngeal nerve as it emerges from the side of the medulla, as first advocated by Dandy (1927), and including the uppermost rootlets of

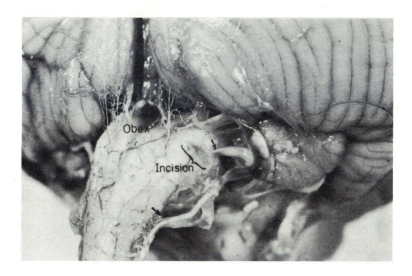

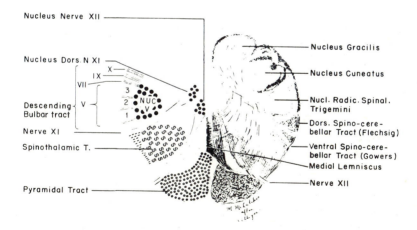

Figure 5.4   The descending bulbar pain tract. Above. Postmortem view of brain stem on elevating cerebellar hemispheres. This shows location of incision caudad to lower end of fourth ventricle (obex). Line of emergence of spinal accessory rootlets marks ventral extent of tractotomy. Below. Transverse section of medulla showing descending sensory fibers of V, VII, IX and X cranial nerves in relation to nuclei of posterior columns and emerging rootlets of spinal accessory nerve.

From J. C. White and W. H. Sweet, *Pain and the Neurosurgeon*, 1969. By courtesy of Charles C. Thomas, Publisher, Springfield, Illinois.

the vagus. The position of these roots is illustrated in Figure 5.2.

2. By incising the dorsomedial portion of the descending bulbar tract, which lies between nucleus cuneatus and the trigeminal fibers, as illustrated in Figure 5.4. Here the pain conducting axones of nervus intermedius, IXth and Xth cranial nerves run in a small, compact bundle. This can be demarcated in the awakened patient by pricking with a pin.

Dr Sweet and I have preferred to cut the glossopharyngeal and uppermost two or three vagal rootlets, having the patient awake to prevent injury to the more caudal motor rootlets which innervate the larynx by stopping at the first sign of hoarseness. The importance of including the uppermost sensory rootlets of the vagus is shown statistically by the fact that in 72 reported patients in whom rhizotomy was limited to the glossopharyngeal nerve one-third suffered subsequent attacks, whereas in the 4 subjects in whom we also cut the uppermost rootlets of the vagus there was no recurrence.

Results

In competent hands complications have been rare, but recurrences are frequent unless the upper vagal rootlets were included in the rhizotomy. We have hesitated to divide the descending bulbar tract because of uncertainty of the level to which these fibers descend. If the tract is cut above the lower end of the fourth ventricle, the patient may be left with an ataxic arm or an unsteady gait; if the transection were below this point we had feared that analgesia of the desired extent might not be obtained. Kunc (1965), its chief advocate, has found that the descending tract of the VIIth, IXth and Xth cranial nerves extends caudally as far as the second cervical roots. In his 11 reported cases of tractotomy performed at the first cervical level, all have been relieved of pain in the posterior tongue, throat and ear with only residual analgesia. This has resulted in no neurological sequelae except occasional and barely noticeable analgesia of the mandibular division and parts of the ear. It has also stopped the attacks of cardiac arrhythmia and asystole with convulsions that occasionally accompany the bouts of pain with spread of impulses to the carotid sinus via the nerve of Hering. This should be the preferable method of treatment in cases of bilateral neuralgia.

NERVUS INTERMEDIUS NEURALGIA

Clinical description
The nervus intermedius is a small sensory branch which accompanies the facial nerve and arises from its geniculate ganglion. It also contains secretory fibers which join the great superficial petrosal nerve. From his study of the cutaneous and mucosal eruption which follows herpetic inflammation of the geniculate ganglion Ramsay Hunt (1915) was able to chart its sensory distribution. This includes the central portion of the auricle with its canal and tympanum, as well as an intraoral distribution to the soft palate and anterior tongue. A few cases have been described in which episodic attacks of pain in this distribution have been reproduced by stimulating the nervus intermedius and relieved after it alone was cut. This syndrome is found in young and middle-aged individuals, not frequently in women. These attacks, which are of intolerable intensity, vary from brief paroxysms of pain in the ear to more prolonged attacks lasting for hours. There may be a trigger zone in the aural canal.

Surgical treatment
Since pain referred to the ear may also be carried by the tympanic branch of the glossopharyngeal or the auricular branch of the vagus, the surgeon should stimulate these structures in the posterior fossa and cut the appropriate roots of the IXth and upper rootlets of the Xth if this is necessary; otherwise only nervus intermedius needs to be cut. Aberrant fibers of nervus intermedius may run in the auditory nerve. If its stimulation is painful this nerve must be sacrificed. This has been necessary in 3 of the reported cases. This form of neuralgia can also be treated by transecting the descending tract of the nerve in the medulla.

Results
In our book on pain (White and Sweet, 1969) Dr Sweet has described the 5 cases reported in the literature and added 2 of our own. In these 7 patients section of nervus intermedius alone was effective in 2. In the others it was necessary to sacrifice the VIIIth nerve also in 2, IXth in one, VIIIth, IXth and part of

Xth in another, and to transect the descending bulbar tract in another after neurotomy of nervus intermedius had failed. All of these were relieved over follow-up periods extending from $2\frac{1}{2}$ months to 21 years. The only complications in this series have been facial paresis, transient in 2 and persistent in 1, and the permanent unilateral deafness that has followed the necessary sacrifice of the auditory nerve. In addition, the single patient treated by a descending bulbar tractotomy developed burning paresthesia of the analgesic side of his face. This might have been avoided by using Kunc's selective section of the VIIth, IXth and Xth component of the descending bulbar tract (Kunc, 1965).

PERIODIC MIGRAINOUS NEURALGIA (CLUSTER HEADACHES)

Clinical description
This syndrome, first accurately described by Harris (1926), is probably a variant of migraine and like it caused by dilatation of intracranial arteries. The attacks consist of severe unilateral burning pain in the temple and forehead, most frequently developing at night forcing the victim to walk the floor. The temporal vessels dilate with the pulsating headache. Attacks usually last for several hours and are accompanied by tearing, nasal congestion and flushing of the skin and conjunctiva. The pain may radiate to the lower face, back of head and neck. It may be accompanied by autonomic disturbances such as facial sweating and ptosis with myosis (Horner's sign). After a series of daily recurrences this neuralgia subsides for a long period, only to be followed by another 'cluster'.

Surgical treatment
If these attacks fail to respond to medication, surgical treatment deserves a trial. Gardner *et al.* (1947) concluded that about half would respond to superficial petrosal neurotomy. Of our 9 patients only 1 has had permanent relief; 4 developed recurrences after 18 to 36 months. The others were not benefited. Late recurrences are probably due to nerve regeneration. This is preventable by cutting the nervus intermedius, which carries the afferent fibers from the petrosal nerve via the geniculate

ganglion, as well as its secretory and vasodilator fibers. Although we have not had an opportunity to test this it has been successfully carried out in 2 patients reported to us by Dr Ernest Sachs, Jr. Transection of the dorsomedial portion of the descending bulbar tract, which carries the pain fibers of the lower cranial sensory nerves, should be an alternative solution.

POST-HERPETIC NEURALGIA

Clinical description
Supraorbital neuralgia is not an uncommon affliction in older individuals after shingles. The continuous burning pain frequently leads to narcotic addiction. Since the viral inflammation often involves the trigeminal fibers in the brain stem as well as the Gasserian ganglion, surgical interruption of its sensory root cannot be counted on to bring relief. Persistent pain in a numb face is an added cause of complaint.

Surgical treatment
The best the surgeon can do is to try supraorbital and supratrochlear block with alcohol, or avulsion, and, in the rare successful case, carry out a permanent interruption of the first division if the pain recurs. In our hands this has been successful in 3 out of 8 attempts. Although we have not as yet had an opportunity to test the effect of radiofrequency stimulation of the inhibitor fibers by means of electrode wires implanted on the nerve at the supraorbital notch, this simple tactic deserves a trial.

TEMPORAL ARTERITIS

Clinical description
This can be a cause of persistent severe pain in the temporal area. It may have an acute onset with fever. The arterial branches are thickened and tender. Intracranial arteries may also be involved. Associated with these clinical manifestations there is commonly a hypochromic anemia and moderate leukocytosis, increase in sedimentation rate and in serum α-2 globulin.

Surgical treatment
Resection of the affected arteries is followed by highly successful results. Six of our patients in whom the diagnosis was confirmed microscopically have had effective relief from one to ten years.

ATYPICAL FACIAL NEURALGIA
Continuous pain in the face with no demonstrable organic cause almost never responds to sensory denervation. The problem is only aggravated if the face is made numb and the pain continues. Space does not permit a discussion of differential diagnosis, or possible surgical treatment in the rare favorable case. The interested reader should read Dr Sweet's description in our monograph on pain.

OCCIPITAL NEURALGIA

Clinical description
The pain in the occiput usually extends down the neck and often into the shoulders; at times into the retro-orbital area as well, owing to the close association of the uppermost cervical roots, which carry its afferent impulses, with the descending trigeminal tract. Its ophthalmic component descends as far as the second cervical vertebra. As pointed out by Hunter and Mayfield (1949), the second cervical nerve is vulnerable to torsion injuries. There is often local point tenderness and pain is likely to be increased by hyperextension of the neck. Occipital neuralgia may result from abnormalities at the base of the skull, as in basilar impression, but it most often follows trauma to the head and neck, as in 'whiplash' injury.

Surgical treatment
Although this neuralgia usually subsides with traction or the support of a Thomas collar, it may persist as a severe, incapacitating complaint. When this is the case, especially when there is an upper cervical spondylosis, the surgeon should try injection of the occipital nerves with a local anesthetic. If repeated blocks give transitory relief, a neurectomy of the greater and lesser occipital nerves as they emerge from the muscles at the base of the occiput is worth trying. At the Massachusetts General Hospital this has been useful in 3 out

of 4 trials. If it fails, a posterior rhizotomy of C2 and C3 is the next step, and it is also important to expose the first cervical nerve, as this may have a sensory component. This operation has been successful in both of our patients, followed 4 and 14 years respectively. Mayfield and Hunter have reported success in 11 of their 23 patients, but their relatively high incidence of failure may have resulted because only the second cervical sensory root was cut in a large proportion.

Pain of spinal origin

ARACHNOIDITIS OF CAUDAL ROOTS
Penetrating wounds and other forms of vertebral trauma are often followed by severe persistent pain. This is especially true in injuries of the cauda equina with constrictive arachnoiditis of the spinal roots. In paraplegia from gunshot wounds its incidence amounts to 10% according to Kahn and Peet (1948). Freeman and Heimburger (1947) reported that 45 of their 600 paraplegics required cordotomy for relief. Since these individuals already have paralyzed bladders and loss of sexual function, a bilateral cordotomy does not involve any additional handicap. In our 13 patients submitted to this procedure, 9 had complete and long-lasting benefit. The failures were due either to inadequate analgesia or other factors such as psychoneurosis with added addiction to narcotics or to scarring of the lower end of the spinal cord. In the latter situation cordotomy is rarely effective. Even resection of the scarred segment will fail unless it is possible to excise the entire area of gliosis. The new method of radiofrequency stimulation of the inhibitor fibers in the posterior column of the spinal cord may prove to be a solution here (see p. 151).

LOCAL SCARRING OF SPINAL NERVES
Radicular pain following vertebral fracture or previous spinal surgery without injury to the spinal cord is usually unilateral and caused by adhesions of the pia-arachnoid or epidural scarring. If it cannot be relieved by lysis of the compressed nerves or foramenotomy, a contralateral cordotomy may succeed if the lesion is situated in the lower half of the spine. In our 18 cases in which this procedure was carried out, 10 have

been permanently relieved. One, an African army officer, subsequently became a leader in his country's revolution. All but 2 of the failures had inadequate or late loss of analgesia. In one this occurred after 18 years, but he was again relieved by a secondary cordotomy.

Having become increasingly aware of the late loss of analgesia that occurs in 40% and the devastating dysesthesia that follows some 10% of the cordotomies in long-term survivors, we have made it our recent policy to substitute posterior rhizotomy when pain is limited to one or two spinal dermatomes. This has given effective relief in three recent cervical and thoracic vertebral fractures. It results in permanent sensory loss and far less frequent complications and deserves a trial before resorting to cordotomy.

RESIDUAL PAIN AFTER LUMBAR DISC SURGERY

The commonest cause of persistent incapacitating pain after herniations of lumbar discs have been removed is epidural scarring. This may encase the fifth lumbar or first sacral nerves in their passage between the dura and intervertebral foramen. The syndrome duplicates the original complaints. In our hands simple lysis of the constricted nerve roots has rarely been successful. In the absence of recurrent disc compression or the coexistence of arachnoiditis, cutting the sensory component of a single compressed nerve has been successful in 7 of our 8 trials. When two nerves were enmeshed in epidural scar our initially good results in 4 out of 5 patients have been vitiated by recurrent pain in all but one. The 3 late failures developed after pain-free periods of 8 months to 7 years. In each it was caused by a spreading arachnoiditis which involved the opposite leg and lower sacral nerves. Echols (1969) has recorded successful results in 60% of his cases, but Loeser (1972) and Onofrio and Campa (1972) have had a large proportion of failures. The only other solution for these victims is either cordotomy, with its well known risk of late failure and complications, or implantation of electrodes on the posterior column of Goll for self-stimulation with induced radiofrequency current (see terminal section on surgical technique). Recent application of this method at the Massachusetts General Hospital has been successful in only 15 of 33 attempts, and the period of follow-up has been short.

COCCYGODYNIA

Following fractures of the coccyx and particularly its amputation, pain may continue in the area between the anus and coccyx. This is aggravated by sitting, even with the weight taken off the end of the sacrum by a rubber ring. Relief in these circumstances has been reported by Bohm and Franksson (1959) in 14 of 15 sufferers by removing the roof of the sacral canal and cutting the tiny rootlets of S4 and S5 intradurally. If a vestigial coccygeal root is present this also should be severed. This leaves the patient with intact perineal and genital sensation, as well as normal urinary and anal sphincter control (supplied by S2 and S3). In our limited experience with 2 cases satisfactory results have been obtained.

LIGHTNING CRISIS OF TABES DORSALIS

Although tabes is now rarely seen, its lightning crises still occasionally require relief from the intense pain in the abdomen and legs. Foerster (1927), who had invariably encountered failure after rhizotomy, vagotomy and sympathectomy, was the first to report success by cordotomy. Since these sufferers have nonfunctioning tabetic bladders and little sexual activity, bilateral cordotomy can be carried out without fear of additional functional loss. Of 9 patients, 7 obtained long-lasting relief and were able to regain weight and stop their narcotics (White and Sweet, 1969). There was only a single early failure and one late recurrence after the level of analgesia fell. None suffered any serious complication and two were able to return to work.

POST-HERPETIC NEURALGIA

Since the virus of herpes zoster produces gliotic lesions not only in the posterior spinal root ganglion but often in its entry zone in the spinal cord as well, posterior rhizotomy is likely to fail. This has been demonstrated by the 4 failures in the 5 attempts reported by Onofrio and Campa (1972). There have been only a few reports of success, just as in supraorbital post-herpetic neuralgia. Excision of the scarred area of skin is also seldom successful. On the other hand, cordotomy is an effective means of relieving the intense burning radicular pain that is a permanent affliction in so many old individuals after an attack of shingles. The level of analgesia must be maintained above the affected dermatome. Following 8 of our cordotomies, pain below the mid-thorax was permanently relieved in half (White and Sweet, 1969). Two suffered late recurrences when analgesia faded and in 2 others psychiatric depression made evaluation difficult. With the recent development of posterior column stimulation we have given this alternative method a trial, but without success in the first three attempts.

Neuralgias of peripheral nerves

Any end-bulb neuroma or neuroma-in-continuity may become a source of chronic disabling pain. As Noordenbos (1959) and Weddell *et al.* (1948) have shown, pain is likely to develop whenever there is a relatively greater degeneration of the larger, well myelinated and rapidly conducting axons that conduct tactile and kinesthetic impulses than of the slowly-conducting C fibers that transmit pain. This situation occurs with partial regeneration of a nerve following trauma, after surgical scarring, or nerve suture with incomplete recovery. This section describes these conditions when the lesion is peripheral to the sensory spinal root ganglion.

NEURALGIA FOLLOWING INJURY TO NERVES IN THE EXTREMITIES

Scarring of the digital nerves may result in such a sensitive finger or toe that the extremity is useless. Digital amputation or reamputation of a painful stump at a higher level* fails all too frequently, as does neurolysis or resection of the neuroma. Cutting back the injured nerve proximal to the scar and burying its healthy end in a tunnel drilled in neighboring bone, or encasing it in a short length of thin Silastic tubing have been helpful methods at times (Ducker and Hayes, 1968). If the patient has a cool, cyanotic hand or foot and the pain is made worse by exposure to cold, regional sympathectomy has given permanent relief in 3 of our 4 trials. Its effectiveness can be

---

* Amputation for relief of pain should be avoided, as it often results in a more painful phantom.

tested in advance by temporarily blocking the stellate or lumbar sympathetic ganglia. Sympathectomy is useful in cases of post-traumatic pain of the hand or foot only. When these simple methods fail it may be necessary for the patient to learn to live with his pain, as it is rarely so severe as to require implantation of electrodes for stimulation of the inhibitor fibers or to justify the risks of cordotomy.

NEUROMAS OF LARGER NERVES

Intraneural scarring in a neuroma-in-continuity is another common cause of chronic disabling pain. This may follow incision across the dorsolateral surface of the wrist with injury to the superficial radial nerve. Here again neurolysis has seldom been successful and even proximal neurotomy of the nerve in the upper forearm has failed.

In the case of persistent painful over-response after suture of the median, ulnar or posterior tibial nerve, as a result of which the patient is unable to grasp objects in his hand or bear weight on the sensitive sole, excision of the neuroma-in-continuity, if complete, with resuture may be effective provided there is better sensory recovery. This, of course, is not justifiable when there has been useful motor recovery.

When there has been compression of the ulnar nerve in its epicondylar groove at the elbow, pain in the hypothenar eminence and last one and one-half fingers may be relieved by transplantation of the nerve out of its scarred bed into healthy tissue in the anteromedial forearm. However, this tactic will fail if there is additional intraneural scarring.

Three out of 6 such sufferers have been successfully rehabilitated by cutting the sensory spinal roots of the ulnar nerve. These are usually limited to C8–T2, but our high rate of failure is presumably due to sensory overlap from the lowermost rootlets of C7 as well.

Posterior rhizotomy has been more helpful in a few instances of pain in the lower extremity. Four of our patients had suffered scarring of the lateral femoral cutaneous nerve after excision of bone from the anterior iliac crest or higher retroperitoneal injury where the nerve lies on the quadratus lumborum muscle. Lasting relief was obtained in 3 by posterior rhizotomy of the upper 2 or 3 lumbar nerves. Satisfactory relief followed upper lumbar rhizotomy in a young woman who had developed saphenous neuralgia following removal of a benign tumor from the medial surface of the tibia. Provided one of the four upper lumbar sensory roots that supply position sense in the quadriceps muscle has been left intact, there have been no complaints of buckling of the knee from loss of postural sensibility.

One individual who developed disabling pain in the lower leg and foot following fracture of both bones above the ankle has been submitted to cordotomy after local neurolysis failed. Fortunately her need for narcotics ceased as soon as her pain was relieved, and there has been no loss of analgesia or other complication.

PAINFUL 'ENTRAPMENT' SYNDROMES
These include constriction of the median nerve in the carpal tunnel and the lateral femoral cutaneous where the nerve passes through the narrow angle between the inguinal (Poupart's) ligament and pubic ramus. The tingling paresthesia that awakens the patient with carpal tunnel syndrome at night and the later sensory loss in the first 3 fingers with weakening of the intrinsic muscles of the thumb are relieved after decompression of the nerve by dividing the carpal ligament. Similar treatment is equally effective in meralgia paresthetica, in which tingling and pain are felt in the lateral aspect of the thigh. Here the nerve is compressed by the overlying inguinal ligament, and decompression by cutting the constricting band is usually sufficient to ensure relief. This simple procedure has freed three of our patients of their complaints. If it fails, the nerve should be cut and allowed to retract upwards. In the rare instance of severe intraneural scarring the upper three lumbar sensory roots may be cut.

INTERCOSTAL NEURALGIA
Radicular pain paralleling the course of ribs that have been cut or forcefully retracted in the course of a thoracotomy, or that follows a thoracic contusion, is not an uncommon disabling complaint. Thoracic surgeons have tried proximal intercostal neurotomy to relieve it, but this is seldom effective. Our policy with these sufferers is first to carry out anesthetic blocks

of the irritable nerve, as well as one above and one below it. This is done by inserting needles alongside the spine to the intervertebral foramina under radiographic control. If this gives temporary relief a hemilaminectomy is carried out and the sensory roots of the nerves involved are cut. It is all-important for the neurosurgeon to realize the great extent of sensory root overlap, as demonstrated by Sherrington in the 1890s (1940) and Foerster (1933) and to cut not only the roots of the involved nerves, but in addition 2 above and below. No patient has complained of the resultant numbness of the thoracic wall, even when 8 roots have been sacrificed. Of 7 patients, 4 have had long-term relief. In one of our failures only 2 sensory roots were cut, and 2 others, after inadequate rhizotomy, have been relieved by additional section of over-lapping roots. Residual overlap can be tested by preliminary diagnostic blocking and by root stimulation in the awakened patient. Loeser (1972), as well as Onofrio and Campa (1972), who have done less extensive rhizotomies, have reported infre-quent success. When properly performed, posterior rhizotomy, with its absence of sensory recovery and fewer complications, gives a better chance of success than cordotomy.

Although I have had no personal experience with per-cutaneous stimulation with the radiofrequency current over an irritated nerve, this new method, described on page 151 deserves a preliminary trial. If successful it can be made more effective by implantation of the electrode on the posterior column for induced transcutaneous stimulation.

NEURALGIAS FOLLOWING MAJOR AMPUTATIONS
Amputation may lead to a persistently tender stump or a painful phantom. In some victims pain is so severe that it leads to total incapacity with narcotic addiction and serious mental depression. In these circumstances radical surgery may be the only means of rehabilitation.

Local pain in the stump
When there is a palpable sensitive neuroma and pain can be stopped by injecting it with anesthetic solution, resection is worth trying once. Injecting the cut central end of the nerve with a neurotoxic solution is not worth while (Guttmann and

Medawar, 1942), but there is evidence that covering it with a short length of thin Silastic rubber tubing is helpful (Ducker and Hayes, 1968). When there are no important muscular branches for some distance above, a proximal neurotomy has been helpful on occasion. One elderly diabetic with severe coronary disease and a tender peroneal neuroma in his below-knee stump, who was well on the road to narcotic addiction, remained pain free for the remaining three years of his life after this procedure.

When these measures fail, radiofrequency stimulation — either percutaneously or by direct implantation of the elec- trodes on the affected nerve — deserves a trial, although our results to date at the Massachusetts General Hospital have not been impressive. The principle of this tactic is fundamentally similar to Ritchie Russell's (1949) suggestion of having the patient pound his sensitive neuroma. Results with posterior column stimulation have been favorable in 5 of 8 trials.

Cordotomy should be resorted to only in desperation, especially in amputations of the arm.

Phantom pain

Henderson and Smyth (1948) have given one of the best accounts of painful phantoms following amputation from their experience with Allied amputees in German prison camps. Although doubted by some, Riddoch's (1948), Falconer's (1954) and our experiences with cordotomy have proved that even if the phantom element is not altered the pain is relieved as long as there is an adequate level of analgesia. In our 18 cases of intolerable phantoms in the lower extremity all but one were freed of discomfort at first, but 6 developed recurrences *pari passu* with partial loss of analgesia. Postcordotomy dys- esthesia was an annoying complication in 3 of these patients.

Although cordotomy was at first equally effective in pain- ful arm phantoms, 3 of our 4 patients eventually suffered recurrences; one after three years of adequate analgesia. Falconer (1954), however, has reported long lasting relief after 4 of his 6 trials.

In this situation implantation of electrodes for radio- frequency stimulation of the posterior column (tractus cuneatus or gracilis) has given good relief in 2 of 4 attempts.

CAUSALGIA AND ALLIED CONDITIONS

The agonizing burning pain that may follow penetrating wounds with a lateral neuroma of one of the major nerves in the arm or leg was first mentioned by Paget in 1864. Later in the same year it was described in greater detail by Mitchell, Morehouse and Keen and named causalgia by Mitchell because of its burning quality. No treatment was known for this intense diffuse burning sensation, aggravated by emotion or exposure to extremes of heat and cold, until Spurling (1930) and Kwan (1935) reported success following sympathectomy. This was confirmed by Doupe, Cullen and Chance (1944) and many others during World War II and the French colonial wars (White and Sweet, 1969). White and Selverstone (1956) had the opportunity to examine 66 veterans a decade later for our Veterans Administration report on nerve injuries. It was then evident that a properly executed sympathetic denervation was nearly always successful. The patients might still have some of the other residual complaints that follow nerve recovery, such as painful over-response or sensitivity to cold, but their disabling burning pain never recurred and all were leading normal lives. For brachial causalgia it is necessary to remove only the second and third thoracic ganglia, thus avoiding the minor annoyance of a Horner's syndrome. After injury to the tibial or peroneal nerves ganglionectomy of L_2 and L_3 should suffice, but with high sciatic involvement it is safer to include the first lumbar and twelfth thoracic ganglia as well.

The efficacy of sympathectomy is best explained by the theory of Doupe *et al.* (1944), further corroborated by Nathan (1947), that sympathetic efferent impulses mediating vaso-constriction, sudo- and pilomotor activity, short-circuit in the area of demyelinization to the afferent somatic pain-conducting axones at the level of injury. Electrical stimulation of the stellate and upper lumbar sympathetic ganglia in conscious patients has shown that the sympathetic is not an accessory pathway for pain from the extremities. Stimulation evokes pain in the extremities only in patients with causalgia (Walker and Nulsen, 1948; White and Sweet, 1969).

Post-traumatic dystrophy following trauma to the hand or foot is another condition which, like causalgia, can be relieved by regional sympathetic denervation. In this condition, which follows contusion of a joint, the patient complains of diffuse burning dysesthesia, often accompanied by rapid decalcification of bone and glossy skin, which is frequently moist and cyanotic. If stellate or lumbar sympathetic block gives temporary but complete relief, this can be made permanent by sympathectomy. Four of our 5 patients received lasting relief from this treatment; 3 others regained full use of a painful extremity without surgery after the simple procedure of regional ganglionic blocks.

Visceral pain

In contrast to the evidence that sympathetic fibers do not transmit pain from the extremities, it is now established that the cardioaortic and splanchnic nerves are the pathways of visceral sensation. While the internal organs are insensitive to pricking, cutting or burning, they react to such physiological stimuli as distension (Hertz, 1911) and ischemia (Sutton and Lueth, 1930). The axons that transmit visceral sensibility belong to the somatic afferent system. After traversing the visceral plexi and paravertebral sympathetic ganglia they enter the spinal cord over its posterior roots from T_1 down through L_2. Pain from the upper esophagus, trachea and main bronchi is carried in the vagi, and from the bladder, rectum and cervix uteri afferent impulses pass through the inferior hypogastric plexus, and enter the cord over the lower sacral nerves (Learmonth, 1931).

It is important to bear in mind that sympathectomy can relieve pain only as long as the disease is confined within the visceral capsule. It cannot be expected to be effective in malignant conditions invading neighboring structures supplied by somatic nerves.

CARDIOAORTIC PAIN

Early attempts to relieve cardiac pain by stellate ganglionectomy often failed. In addition to the long-known cardiac sympathetic nerves from the three cervical ganglia, smaller thoracic rami were discovered by G. A. G. Mitchell (1956) and others. These were found to contain sensory fibers by the experimental studies of White, Garrey and Atkins (1933). Fortunately this work on the dog has proved applicable to man. Experience has shown that cardiac pain can be relieved consistently either by removing the stellate and upper three thoracic sympathetic ganglia or by cutting the posterior roots from T_1 down through T_4. This has been corroborated in 13 of our patients as well as in 29 others reported in the literature (White and Sweet, 1969). Even though many present-day sufferers from angina decubitus can be relieved by revascularization of the myocardium, cardiac denervation is still useful in the occasional patient when this has failed.

We have similarly been able to stop the continuous pain of rapidly expanding aortic aneurysms by paravertebral infiltration of alcohol around the stellate and second thoracic ganglia in 3 which involved the aortic arch; also in 2 cases of inoperable aneurysms of the thoracic and upper abdominal aorta by posterior rhizotomy (White and Sweet, 1969). Removal of the paravertebral sympathetic ganglia would have been hazardous because of the likelihood of rupturing the aneurysmal sac.

GASTROINTESTINAL PAIN

Postcholecystectomy neuralgia, when due to back-pressure on the biliary ducts, is equally well relieved by splanchnicectomy, provided it responds well to diagnostic block (White *et al.*, 1952). This is necessary to rule out the presence of a painful neuroma in the abdominal incision. At the Massachusetts General Hospital 14 patients have now been treated by splanchnicectomy (White and Sweet, 1969). Only a right-sided operation is necessary when pain is unilateral. Of these patients, 12 have now been relieved by resecting the major and minor splanchnic nerves with the lower three thoracic sympathetic ganglia. One of the 2 failures later turned out to have a penetrating duodenal ulcer.

Relief of the deep aching pain of chronic pancreaticolithiasis is far less successful. Only 3 of 7 patients obtained lasting benefit following splanchnicectomy. The probable explanation of these failures is that the inflammatory process extends beyond the capsule of the gland and thereby involves tissue innervated by intercostal nerves.

In 6 patients complaining of severe intermittent colicky pain due to adhesive bands constricting loops of small bowel after laparotomy, splanchnic block has resulted in the passage of flatus with temporary relief. These subjects all recovered after splanchnicectomy. This operation is based on the experimental work of Bentley and Smithwick (1940), who showed that the midline abdominal distress induced by balloon distension of the small bowel is no longer felt after splanchnicectomy.

Incapacitating nephralgia may follow operations on the kidney. The deep colicky pain in the costophrenic angle radiating to the groin can be relieved surgically. Gunnar Bauer (1944) and others first reported success by stripping the nerves in the vascular pedicle of the kidney. This has been effective in our hands in one case. From his anatomical studies Mitchell (1956) found that this operation cannot be counted on to interrupt all afferent pathways from the kidney. We have therefore preferred to resect portions of the three splanchnic nerves as they pass through the crus of the diaphragm with the adjacent thoracolumbar sympathetic ganglia or to cut the corresponding posterior roots ($T_{9 \text{ or } 10}$–L_2). These operations have proved satisfactory in 3 subjects who subsequently could feel no discomfort on retrograde distension of the renal pelvis. Each subject should first be tested by diagnostic splanchnic block to make certain that the pain is not caused by an incisional neuroma. In that event it is necessary to resort to posterior rhizotomy, which denervates the body wall as well as the kidney and upper ureter. This has relieved two other patients.

IDIOPATHIC DYSMENORRHEA
The excessive suprapubic pain with backache that afflicts some young women at the time of their menses can be relieved in a high proportion of instances by resection of the superior hypogastric plexus (Cotte's operation) (Cotte, 1925). With the recent improvements in hormonal therapy this presacral neurectomy does not require further discussion.

Surgical technique
This section is included in order to give the reader who has no knowledge of neurosurgical technique an understanding of the extent, advantages and risks of the operations in common use for relief of pain. Since these procedures are used in the treat-

ment of pain of cancer as well as the non-malignant neuralgias, it has been agreed to avoid repetition by describing here only those used in treating the cephalalgias, causalgia and visceral disease of non-malignant etiology in this chapter. The techniques of cordotomy and posterior spinal rhizotomy, both surgical and chemical, are discussed in Chapter 6.

RETROGASSERIAN RHIZOTOMY

Subtemporal operation [*Frazier's technique*] (Frazier, 1925)
This approach to the Gasserian ganglion is illustrated in Figure 5.1. It is carried out under intratracheal anesthesia with the patient sitting and the long axis of the head fixed at 90° to the surgeon's line of vision. Only a small craniectomy is required in the thin lower portion of the temporal bone. The dura is then elevated from the base of the skull. After coagulation of the middle meningeal artery, this is severed at its exit from the foramen spinosum. The foramen is packed with a wisp of cotton to prevent possible bleeding. The temporal lobe dura is then peeled off the base of the skull, extending the dissection medially and posteriorly to the foramen ovale and the Gasserian ganglion, which lies just behind. The dissection should be carried back to the tip of the petrous ridge in order to obtain a good exposure of the root sheath in Meckel's cave. This contains the trigeminal fibers floating in cerebrospinal fluid. After the root sheath has been opened the desired portion of the sensory rootlets is elevated on a nerve hook and cut. Care must be taken to find and preserve the motor rootlet which runs obliquely downward behind the sensory fascicles to enter the foramen ovale. In order to avoid regeneration it is important to cut the sensory fibers several millimeters behind the ganglion.

An alternative to cutting the sensory rootlets is to compress them with moderate force by pressure of a cotton pledget, as described by Shelden (1966). This usually spares the patient the annoyance of total anesthesia and greatly reduces the complications of disagreeable paresthesia and keratitis.

As pointed out above (see Table 5.1), retrogasserian rhizotomy carries very little risk of mortality. Its major handicap is disagreeable paresthesias or anesthesia dolorosa in the anesthetic area. It is important to preserve the motor root and, whenever possible, the fibers of the first division in order to avoid complicating keratitis. Loss of vision can usually be prevented by temporary suture of the eyelids.

Suboccipital operation [*Dandy's technique*] (Dandy, 1937)
The posterior approach to the trigeminal nerve as it emerges from the pons to cross the petrous ridge and enter Meckel's cave is illustrated in Figure 5.2. The operation is done with the patient seated and head rigidly secured in maximum flexion. After making a long paramedian incision from the level of the inion to the spinous process of the second cervical vertebra, the surgeon divides and retracts the occipitospinal muscles. Then the thin occipital bone is removed from the midline out to the mastoid, the dura opened and hinged back laterally. This exposes the cerebellar hemisphere and its tonsil, which are retracted medially. After the arachnoid has been opened and the cisterna magna drained, the seventh and eighth nerves are seen as they leave the upper medulla and enter the acoustic meatus. The exposure must then be carried upward into the cerebellopontine angle, taking care not to injure the posterior-inferior cerebellar artery. With a lighted retractor the fifth nerve can be exposed as it approaches the petrous ridge to enter its root sleeve in Meckel's cave. It is of the greatest importance to search for and, if necessary, to coagulate the petrosal vein, which usually crosses the nerve root at this point. Once this is done the entire bundle of sensory fibers can be cut without fear of damaging the motor division. This emerges from the pons more rostrally.

This operation is more difficult and somewhat more hazardous than the subtemporal approach. With the exception of sparing the motor root, its only advantage is the occasional discovery of a tumor or aneurysm compressing the nerve, and its value in cases of malignant disease in which other sensory roots must be cut in addition for the relief of pain in the throat and ear.

GLOSSOPHARYNGEAL AND
UPPER VAGAL RHIZOTOMY
Experience has taught us that to ensure certain relief of so-

called glossopharyngeal neuralgia the upper vagal rootlets must be included in the rhizotomy. These often carry overlapping sensory fibers. This operation should be performed in the horizontal lateral cerebellar position, so that cerebrospinal fluid will not drain off and produce intense headache when the patient is awakened for testing.

Using the approach illustrated in Figure 5.2, it is easy to find the IXth and Xth nerves as they emerge from the medulla and pass laterally to the jugular foramen. They enter the foramen just above the spinal accessory nerve. The posterior-inferior cerebellar artery lies adjacent to these structures and must be protected. After the large fascicle of the glossopharyngeal has been cut the patient should be awakened. It is then possible to stimulate the upper vagal rootlets in turn and to cut the uppermost two or three that give rise to a painful response. Great care must be taken to stop at the first trace of hoarseness of the voice.

Since we have taken to cutting the uppermost vagal rootlets there have been no recurrences of neuralgia, formerly a common complication when rhizotomy was limited to the glossopharyngeal root. Any resultant hoarseness has rapidly cleared. There should be no significant muscular weakness or postoperative paresthesia, and the sensory loss is not a cause for complaint.

RHIZOTOMY OF NERVUS INTERMEDIUS
In cases of neuralgia referred to the ear it must be borne in mind that this area is innervated by the Vth, IXth and Xth cranial nerves, and also by the nervus intermedius, the sensory division of the VIIth. In addition to its gustatory fibers (via the chorda tympani from the lingual nerve) and secretory fibers (via the greater superficial petrosal and vidian nerve to the sphenopalatine ganglion) the intermedius carries sensory afferents from the skin around the aural canal and middle ear, as well as from the mucous membrane near the tonsil. Sensory fibers also enter its geniculate ganglion via the greater superficial petrosal nerve (White and Sweet, 1969). It is important to remember that pain deep in the ear may be transmitted over the glossopharyngeal or vagus as well as the nervus intermedius. The only way to determine with certainty the pathway

is to awaken the patient at operation and stimulate these nerves in the posterior fossa.

The intermedius consists of a tiny bundle of fibers lying on the posterior surface of the facial nerve. At times it runs in the acoustic, so if it is not found in its usual position this nerve should be stimulated and, if necessary, cut. Unilateral deafness is a fair price to pay for relief of intolerable aural neuralgia. Intermedius neurotomy has also been used by Sachs (1968) for the relief of periodic migrainous neuralgia (cluster headaches).

The intermedius is exposed by the suboccipital route shown in Figure 5.2. It is brought into view by gently depressing the acoustic nerve and thus uncovering the posterior surface of the facial (Figure 5.2, C).

Following neurotomy the patient should suffer no annoying complications beyond loss of taste on the side of the tongue. Spontaneous tearing is also abolished, but normal moisture of the conjunctival surface is preserved.

CHEMICAL OR THERMAL COAGULATION OF GASSERIAN GANGLION AND ITS ROOT FIBERS

With radiographic control, insertion of a needle for injection of neurotoxic agents or electrocoagulation of the Gasserian ganglion and its root fibers in Meckel's cave is a simple procedure in the hands of an experienced operator. The needle is inserted through the skin 2.5–3 cm lateral to the labial commissure and guided through the cheek with the help of a finger in the mouth. It is aimed at the ipsilateral lacrimal caruncle and a point is marked on the zygoma 3–4 cm in front of the aural canal. Checking with x-ray films greatly facilitates its insertion through the foramen ovale. The needle is shown in lateral projection in Figure 5.3. Here the tip has been advanced to the extreme end of the root sleeve, 5 mm behind the profile of the clivus. This is too deep for safe injection and with coagulation is likely to result in loss of the corneal reflex. It should be withdrawn to a point close to the anterior surface of the clivus. At this depth cerebrospinal fluid should still be obtained on removing the stylet.

With the patient lying on his back and the head tilted backward so that the needle is pointed directly downward, hypobaric alcohol, injected in tiny increments, becomes trapped within the root sheath. If hyperbaric phenol in glycerine is used, the injection is performed with the patient seated and the head flexed forward, so that the needle is pointed directly upward.

When Sweet and Wepsic's (1974) technique of heating the uninsulated tip of the needle by radiofrequency current is employed the electrode should be inserted to a point just behind the profile of the clivus for relief of first and second division pain; and to just short of the clivus for pain in the second and third divisions. By manipulation of its tip into the superior-medial or inferior-lateral portion of the root fibers pain on electrical stimulation should be evoked in the area of first and second or second and third divisions. When the surgeon is satisfied that the electrode is correctly placed, a thermister tip to control the degree of heating is inserted through the needle. Brief acting anesthesia is then induced by intravenous Brevital (methohexital) and the tip heated to 50–70 °C by radiofrequency current over a period of 50 seconds. The patient is then awakened so that the extent and degree of sensory loss can be tested. If not satisfactory it can be increased by repeating the procedure and heating up to 100 °C. The goal is to limit sensory loss to high-grade hypalgesia in the desired portion of the face, with preservation of tactile sensibility and the corneal reflex.

This promises to be the ideal method for surgical treatment of *tic douloureux*. It requires only an overnight hospitalization. Since sensory loss need not be carried to the stage of numbness, disagreeable paresthesia is a rare complication. The corneal reflex can usually be preserved, thus nearly eliminating the risk of keratitis. There has been no lasting paralysis of the motor root or other cranial nerves in over 300 trials.

TRACTOTOMY OF DESCENDING FIBERS OF Vth, VIIth, IXth AND Xth CRANIAL NERVES

This operation was proposed by Sjöqvist (1938) as a method of relieving trigeminal neuralgia with the preservation of tactile and postural sensibility*. Subsequently it was found to

---

* Only the axons conducting pain and thermal discrimination run in the descending root. Those which transmit tactile and postural sensibility enter the main sensory nucleus in the upper medulla.

interrupt pain conduction in the nervus intermedius, glosso-pharyngeus and vagus as well (Brodal, 1947; White and Sweet, 1969). In the medulla at the level of the lower end of the fourth ventricle (obex) this tract lies between the nuclei of the posterior columns and the emerging rootlets of the spinal accessory nerve (Figure 5.4A). The spinothalamic tract is just ventral. The pain-conducting fibers of trigeminus are situated ventrally and the more compact bundle of fibers from nervus intermedius, glossopharyngeus and vagus in its most dorsal portion (Kunc, 1965) (Figure 5.4B).

Tractotomy is carried out under short-acting general anesthesia with the patient in the lateral cerebellar position. It is important not to elevate the head, so that cerebrospinal fluid cannot run off and produce an intense headache, as the patient must be awakened to test the extent of analgesia. Only a small amount of occipital bone is removed along with the rim of the foramen magnum and arch of the Atlas vertebra. After opening the dura and retracting the cerebellar tonsil the surgeon has a good view of the lower medulla and uppermost segment of the spinal cord (Figure 5.4A). For relief of trigeminal pain an incision is made at the level of or just below the obex, the blade being inserted at the level of the emerging spinal-accessory rootlets. This is carried to a depth of 3 mm and swept dorsally into the lateral edge of nucleus cuneatus. The patient is then awakened to be tested for the extent of analgesia. In cases of neuralgia involving nervus intermedius, glossopharyngeus and vagus the position of their pain-conducting fibers can be localized by pricking the medulla of the awakened patient with a pin, as described by Falconer (1954) and Kunc (1965). The location of these components of the tract is illustrated in Figure 5.4B). All but the mandibular fibers of trigeminus, which terminate just below the obex, descend at least as far as the first cervical segment of the cord. If the incision is made more rostrally the patient may develop ataxia of the arm or lateral deviation of gait. Kunc (personal communication) has now been able to relieve the pain of glossopharyngeal-vagal neuralgia in 11 subjects by a selective transection of the dorsomedial portion of the descending tract with preservation of normal sensation in the face except in the area supplied by the mandibular division.

Tractotomy is a valuable procedure to perform on one side in cases of bilateral trigeminal neuralgia. It is useful for the relief of neuralgia of nervus intermedius when this is not obtained by rhizotomy, as well as in periodic migrainous neuralgia ('cluster headache'). It is also an alternative method (preferred by Kunc, 1965) in cases of glossopharyngeal-vagal neuralgia.

SYMPATHECTOMY

Removal of portions of the chain of paravertebral sympathetic ganglia or splanchnic nerves is a most useful procedure for relieving persistent pain in visceral disease or causalgia. To be effective for the former, disease must be confined within the visceral capsule, as in angina pectoris, aortic aneurysm, post-cholecystectomy or postoperative renal pain. When malignant disease has spread beyond the confines of the visceral capsule, sympathectomy is usually ineffective because of involvement of somatic nerves in the retroperitoneal tissues. Sympathectomy is also nearly always successful in the relief of causalgia from penetrating wounds of nerves or in the post-traumatic dystrophies that follow trauma to joints with diffuse pain and trophic changes. Its effectiveness can readily be predicted by temporarily blocking the regional sympathetic ganglia or splanchnic nerves by paravertebral injection of local anesthetic solutions.

The pathways of visceral pain from the peripheral plexuses through the cardiac and splanchnic nerves, paravertebral ganglia, rami communicantes, spinal nerves and their posterior sensory roots are illustrated in Figure 5.5. Anatomical details of these connections are well described in Mitchell's (1965) textbook. It should be pointed out that all the sensory fibers from the cardioaortic and upper abdominal viscera funnel into the spinal cord between its first thoracic and second lumbar segment. Pain from the bladder cannot be relieved by sympathectomy, as it enters the sacral portion of the cord. The vagi transmit sensation only from the upper esophagus, trachea and bronchi.

Upper thoracic sympathetic ganglionectomy — The stellate and upper three thoracic ganglia are situated at the junction of the three upper ribs with the sides of the corresponding vertebrae.

VISCUS	SEGMENTAL INNERVATIONS	NERVES	PLEXUSES

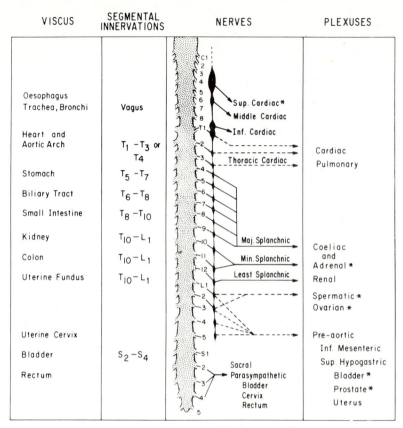

Oesophagus Trachea, Bronchi	Vagus	Sup. Cardiac* Middle Cardiac	
Heart and Aortic Arch	$T_1 - T_3$ or T_4	Inf. Cardiac Thoracic Cardiac	Cardiac Pulmonary
Stomach	$T_5 - T_7$		
Biliary Tract	$T_6 - T_8$		
Small Intestine	$T_8 - T_{10}$		
Kidney	$T_{10} - L_1$	Maj. Splanchnic	Coeliac and Adrenal*
Colon	$T_{10} - L_1$	Min. Splanchnic	
Uterine Fundus	$T_{10} - L_1$	Least Splanchnic	Renal
			Spermatic* Ovarian*
Uterine Cervix			Pre-aortic Inf. Mesenteric
Bladder	$S_2 - S_4$		Sup. Hypogastric
Rectum		Sacral Parasympathetic Bladder Cervix Rectum	Bladder* Prostate* Uterus

* No known sensory fibers in sympathetic rami

From J. C. White and W. H. Sweet, *Pain and the Neurosurgeon*, 1969. By courtesy of Charles C. Thomas, Publisher, Springfield, Illinois.

They lie just ventral to the point where the intercostal nerves enter their intervertebral foramina and are connected to these nerves by their communicant rami. Depending on the surgeon's experience, ganglionectomy can be carried out either by:

1. Adson's posterior approach after resecting the central end of the second rib (Adson, 1931).

2. Gask's supraclavicular approach after cutting the insertion of scalenus anticus muscle and following the subclavian artery down to the origin of the vertebral. The stellate ganglion lies just behind this point (Gask, 1933).

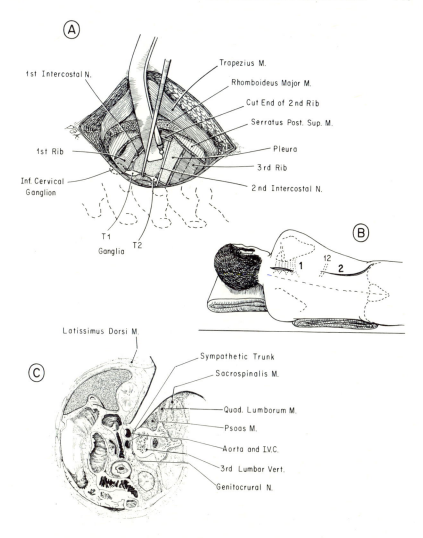

Figure 5.6 Thoracic and lumbar sympathetic ganglionectomy. A. Resection of stellate and upper thoracic ganglia after excision of central end of second rib. B. Location of incisions for resection of: 1. Upper thoracic ganglia. 2. Upper lumbar ganglia. C. Position of lumbar ganglionated chain.

3. The axillary transcostal approach through the pleura by which the apex of the lung can be retracted to expose the paravertebral chain at the sides of the upper thoracic vertebrae.

To relieve cardiac pain the entire stellate down through the third thoracic ganglion must be removed (Figure 5.6A). In causalgia it is only necessary to resect the second and third ganglia, which usually spares the subject the disfigurement of a drooping upper eyelid and constricted pupil (Horner's sign).

Lumbar sympathetic ganglionectomy — The chain of lumbar ganglia runs along the anterolateral aspect of the vertebrae between the aorta or vena cava and the medial border of the psoas muscle (Figure 5.6C). The upper lumbar chain is brought into view by cutting through the fascia between the quadratus lumborum and abdominal muscles, then separating the renal capsule and peritoneum off the quadratus lumborum and psoas muscle.

For relief of causalgia and post-traumatic dystrophy the second and third lumbar ganglia should be removed, carrying the excision upward through the crus of the diaphragm in patients with high sciatic scarring.

Splanchnicectomy — For relief of postcholecystectomy neuralgia or colicky pain from distension of loops of small bowel caused by adhesions after laparotomy, resection of the major splanchnic nerve and lower thoracic ganglia is usually very effective. This supradiaphragmatic sympathectomy is carried

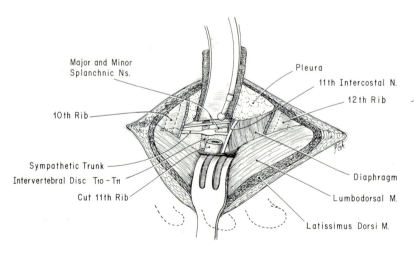

Figure 5.7   Splanchnicectomy through eleventh rib incision.

out through a central resection of the eleventh rib (Figure 5.7). It is wise to test by a preoperative splanchnic block to make sure that the pain can be totally relieved. This operation often fails in cases of chronic pancreaticolithiasis, presumably because the inflammatory process has extended beyond the glandular capsule. In cases of postoperative nephralgia it is necessary to include the minor and least splanchnic nerves and to carry the ganglionectomy down through the diaphragm to include the first lumbar ganglion. This necessitates resection of the twelfth rib.

It is of interest to point out the effectiveness of sympathectomy, as well as its freedom from serious complications. In a personal series of 67 subjects operated upon for visceral pain 87% have been relieved over periods up to 22 years; of 14 patients with causalgia operated upon in Naval hospitals during World War II, all have maintained long-lasting relief of their intense and totally disabling burning dysesthesia. In a series of 66 patients examined with Selverstone (White and Selverstone, 1956) for our Veterans Administration, all who had had an adequate sympathectomy had maintained their initial freedom from burning pain over a period of many years. These excellent results are similar to those described by British surgeons and the experience of the French in their colonial wars.

ACTIVATION OF INHIBITOR FIBERS

A recently developed method of relieving pain due to gliotic lesions in peripheral nerves or the spinal cord is electrical stimulation of the heavily myelinated, rapidly conducting A fibers. This can inhibit the more slowly transmitted, painful impulses in the smaller, unmyelinated C fibers. Inhibition is controlled by the 'gate mechanism' described by Melzack and Wall (1965). Clinical application was first described by Sweet (White and Sweet, 1969) and its adaptation to the posterior spinal columns advocated by Shealy (see Burton, 1973).

Stimulation is carried out by means of electrodes placed on the skin over the affected nerve trunk or implanted directly on the peripheral nerve or the posterior column (tractus gracilis or cuneatus). In the case of deep implantation the electrodes are connected by fine insulated wires to an induction coil buried beneath the skin. The inhibitor fibers can thus be stimulated by induced radiofrequency current by means of a small battery operated generator placed over the subcutaneous receiving coil. The current is increased to the point which produces a mild tingling in the painful area. In favorable cases the patient can obtain rapid relief whenever his pain becomes intolerable. This is often maintained for increasingly prolonged periods.

The handicaps with this method are the proper placement of the electrodes so that paresthesia is induced in the painful area; also the subsequent mechanical difficulties in maintaining electrode contact. The details of the apparatus and the parameters of current are described in a recent report of Sweet and Wepsic (in press) and that of Burton (1973) on a seminar on dorsal column stimulation.

Table 5.2 EARLY RESULTS OF RADIOFREQUENCY STIMULATION OF THE POSTERIOR COLUMNS

Cause of pain	Total cases	Satisfactory relief	Partial relief	Failure
SPINAL CORD				
Trauma	4		1	3
Post-operation for tumor	1			1
Post-operation for A–V anomaly	1			1
Post-cordotomy dysesthesia	7	2	1	4
Post-meningitis	1			1
Post-irradiation	3		1	2
Multiple sclerosis	3	1		2
SPINAL NERVE ROOTS				
Post-herpetic	3			3
Post-operative adhesions, epidural and intra-arachnoid:				
Cervical	7	4		3
Lumbar	33	5	10	18
Avulsion of brachial plexus	1	1		
Post-rhizotomy dysesthesia	1	1		
PERIPHERAL NERVES				
Neuromas	7	2	2	3
Amputation stump	8	2	3	3
Phantom limb	4	1	1	2
Post-infectious	2	1		1
Totals:	86	20	19	47

Results of posterior column stimulation at the Massachusetts General Hospital at the hands of Sweet and Wepsic, not yet published, are summarized in Table 5.2. They have not yet compiled statistics on percutaneous or direct stimulation of peripheral nerves. Other statistics from Dr Shealy's clinic are included in Burton's report. While this innocuous method deserves widespread trial, it has not yet reached the stage of consistent success nor has sufficient experience accumulated to draw valid conclusions on its ultimate value.

Conclusions
Analysis of the statistics reported in this chapter shows that much still remains to be learned to improve the effectiveness of relieving uncontrollable chronic pain by surgery. Nature, given time, has an extraordinary ability to find new pathways for conducting pain. At times unexpected and most unpleasant complaints have developed. However, the results in over 9,000 patients included in this report show that nearly 80% have obtained worthwhile results. Although the relief of suffering and ultimate psychological deterioration that follows prolonged incapacity and dependence on narcotics often rewards the surgeon's efforts, more consistently effective and safer methods remain to be developed. Provided the effectiveness of stimulating the pain-inhibitor fibers can be improved, this goal may come within our reach.

Acknowledgement
I am indebted to Drs William H. Sweet and James G. Wepsic for giving me their most recent statistics on electrical coagulation of the trigeminal root fibers and on activation of the pain inhibitor axons by radiofrequency stimulation. In addition I particularly want to thank Mr Antony Jefferson for his kindness in reading the text and assuring me that my descriptions of these neuralgias and surgical procedures for their relief are in agreement with current views of British neurological surgeons.

REFERENCES

Adson, A. W. (1931). Cervicothoracic ganglionectomy, trunk resection, and rami-sectomy by the posterior intrathoracic approach. *Amer. J. Surg.*, *11*, 227

Bauer, G. (1944). Late results of denervation of the kidney for renal pain. *Acta Chir. Scand.*, *90*, 460

Bentley, F. H. and Smithwick, R. H. (1940). Visceral pain produced by balloon distension of the jejunum. *Lancet*, *239*, 389

Bohm, E. and Franksson, C. (1959). Coccygodynia and sacral rhizotomy. *Acta Chir. Scand.*, *116*, 268

Brodal, A. (1947). Central course of afferent fibers for pain in facial, glossopharyngeal and vagus nerves: Clinical observations. *A.M.A. Arch. Neurol. Psychiat.*, *57*, 292

Burton, C. (1973). Seminar on dorsal column stimulation: Summary of proceedings, Temple University Sugarloaf Conference Center, September 23, 1972. *Surg. Neurol.*, *1*, 285

Cotte, G. (1925). Sur le traitement des dysménorrhées rebelles par la sympathectomie hypogastrique périartérielle ou la section du nerf présacré. *Lyon Med.*, *135*, 153

Dandy, W. E. (1927). Glossopharyngeal neuralgia (tic douloureux); its diagnosis and treatment. *A.M.A. Arch. Surg.*, *15*, 198

Doupe, J., Cullen, C. H. and Chance, G. Q. (1944). Post-traumatic pain and the causalgic syndrome. *J. Neurol. Neurosurg. Psychiat.*, *7*, 33

Ducker, T. B. and Hayes, G. J. (1968). Experimental improvements in the use of silastic cuff for peripheral nerve repair. *J. Neurosurg. 28*, 582

Echols, D. H. (1969). Sensory rhizotomy following operation for ruptured inter-vertebral disc. A review of 62 cases. *J. Neurosurg.*, *31*, 335

Falconer, M. A. (1953). Surgical treatment of intractable phantom-limb pain. *Brit. Med. J.*, *1*, 299

Falconer, M. A. (1954). First and second division trigeminal neuralgia treated by intramedullary trigeminal tractotomy. *Proc. Roy. Soc. Med.*, *47*, 299

Foerster, O. (1927). *Die Leitungsbahnen des Schmerzgefühls und die chirurgische Behandlung der Schmerzzustände.* Berlin: Urban & Schwarzenberg, 360 pp.

Foerster, O. (1933). The dermatomes in man. *Brain*, *56*, 1

Frazier, C. H. (1925). Subtotal resection of sensory root for relief of major trigeminal neuralgia. *A.M.A. Arch. Neurol. Psychiat.*, *13*, 378

Freeman, L. W. and Heimburger, R. F. (1947). Surgical relief of pain in paraplegic patients. *A.M.A. Arch. Surg.*, *55*, 433

Gardner, W. J., Stowell, A. and Dutlinger, R. (1947). Resection of the greater super-ficial petrosal nerve in the treatment of unilateral headache. *J. Neurosurg.*, *4*, 105

Gask, G. E. (1933). The surgery of the sympathetic nervous system. *Brit. J. Surg.*, *21*, 113

Guttmann, L. and Medawar, P. B. (1942). The chemical inhibition of fiber regenera-tion and neuroma formation in peripheral nerves. *J. Neurol. Neurosurg. Psychiat.*, *5*, 130

Harris, W. (1926). *Neuritis and Neuralgia.* London: Oxford University Press, 418 pp.

Harris, W. (1940). An analysis of 1,433 cases of paroxysmal trigeminal neuralgia (trigeminal-tic) and the end-results of gasserian alcohol injection. *Brain*, *63*, 209

Henderson, W. R. and Smyth, G. E. (1948). Phantom limbs. *J. Neurol. Neurosurg. Psychiat.*, N.S. *11*, 88

Hertz, A. F. (1911). On the sensibility of the alimentary canal in health and disease. *Lancet*, *1*, 1051

Hunt, J. R. (1915). The sensory field of the facial nerve: A further contribution to the symptomatology of the geniculate ganglion. *Brain*, *38*, 418

Hunter, C. R. and Mayfield, F. H. (1949). Role of the upper cervical roots in the production of pain in the head. *Amer. J. Surg.*, *78*, 743

Jaeger, R. (1959). The results of injecting hot water into the Gasserian ganglion for the relief of tic douloureux. *J. Neurosurg.*, *16*, 656

Jefferson, A. (1966). Trigeminal neuralgia: Trigeminal root and ganglion injections using phenol in glycerin. In: Knighton, R. S. and Dumke, P. R. (eds.). *Pain*. Henry Ford Hospital International Symposium. Boston: Little, Brown & Co., pp. 365–371

Kahn, E. A. and Peet, M. M. (1948). The technique of anterolateral cordotomy. *J. Neurosurg.*, *5*, 276

Kunc, Z. (1965). Treatment of essential neuralgia of the 9th nerve by selective tractotomy. *J. Neurosurg.*, *23*, 494

Kwan, S. T. (1935). The treatment of causalgia by thoracic sympathetic ganglionectomy. *Ann. Surg.*, *101*, 222

Learmonth, J. R. (1931). Neurosurgery in the treatment of diseases of the urinary bladder. II. Treatment of vesical pain. *J. Urol.*, *26*, 13

Loeser, J. D. (1972). Dorsal rhizotomy for the relief of chronic pain. *J. Neurosurg.*, *36*, 745

Mayfield, F. and Hunter, C. (1952). The role of the cervical roots in the production of pain in the head and face. Presented at the 14th annual meeting of the American Academy of Neurological Surgery, New York, October 1, 1952

Melzack, R. and Wall, P. D. (1965). Pain mechanisms: A new theory. *Science*, *150*, 971

Mitchell, G. A. G. (1956). *Cardiovascular Innervation*. Edinburgh & London: Livingstone, 356 pp.

Mitchell, S. W., Morehouse, G. R. and Keen, W. W., Jr. (1864). *Gunshot Wounds and Other Injuries of Nerves*. Philadelphia: J. B. Lippincott & Co., 164 pp.

Nathan, P. W. (1947). On the pathogenesis of causalgia in peripheral nerve injuries. *Brain*, *70*, 145

Noordenbos, W. (1959). *Pain. Problems Pertaining to the Transmission of Nerve Impulses Which Give Rise to Pain. Preliminary Statement*. Amsterdam: Elsevier Publishing Co., 182 pp.

Onofrio, B. M. and Campa, H. K. (1972). Evaluation of rhizotomy. Review of 12 years' experience. *J. Neurosurg.*, *36*, 751

Paget, J. (1864). Clinical lecture on some cases of local paralysis (delivered at St. Bartholomew's Hospital on February 6, 1864). *Med. Times and Hosp. Gaz.*, *Lond.*, *1*, 331

Penman, J. (1953). Some developments in the technique of trigeminal injection. *Lancet*, *1*, 760

Pudenz, R. H. and Shelden, C. H. (1952). Experiences with foraminal decompression in the surgical treatment of tic douloureux. Presented at the 14th annual meeting of the American Academy of Neurological Surgery, New York, September, 1952

Riddoch, G. (1941). Phantom limbs and body shape. *Brain*, *64*, 197

Russell, W. R. (1949). Painful amputation stumps and phantom limbs. Treatment by repeated percussion to the stump neuromata. *Brit. Med. J.*, *1*, 1024

Sachs, E., Jr. (1968). The role of the nervus intermedius in facial neuralgia. Report of four cases with observations on the pathways for taste, lacrimation and pain in the face. *J. Neurosurg.*, *28*, 54

Shelden, C. H. (1966). Compression procedure for trigeminal neuralgia. *J. Neurosurg.*, *25*, 374

Sherrington, C. S. (1940). On the distribution of the sensory nerve-roots. Ch. II in: Denny-Brown, D. (ed.) *Selected Writings of Sir Charles Sherrington*: New York, Paul B. Hoeber, 532 pp.

Sjöqvist, O. (1938). Eine neue Operationsmethode bei Trigeminusneuralgie: Durchschneidung des Tractus spinalis trigemini. *Zentralbl. Neurochir.*, *2*, 274

Sjöqvist, O. (1949). Surgical section of pain tracts and pathways in the spinal cord and brain stem. *4th International Neurological Congress, Paris*, *1*, 119

Spurling, R. G. (1930). Causalgia of the upper extremity. Treatment by dorsal sympathetic ganglionectomy. *A.M.A. Arch. Neurol. Psychiat.*, *23*, 784

Sweet, W. H. and Wepsic, J. G. (1974). Controlled thermocoagulation of trigeminal ganglion and rootlets for differential destruction of pain fibers. I. Trigeminal neuralgia. *J. Neurosurg.*, in press

Sweet, W. H. and Wepsic, J. G. Electrical stimulation for suppression of pain in man. Presented at Houston Neurologic Symposium, March 1–3, 1973, to be published in *Symposia Specialist*

Sutton, D. C. and Lueth, H. C. (1930). Pain. *A.M.A. Arch. Int. Med.*, *45*, 827

Thiry, S. (1962). Expérience personnelle basée sur 225 cas de névralgie essentielle du trijumeau traités par électrocoagulation stéréotaxique du ganglion de Gasser entre 1950 et 1960. *Neurochirurgie*, *8*, 86

Walker, A. E. and Nulsen, F. (1948). Electrical stimulation of the upper thoracic portion of the sympathetic chain in man. *A.M.A. Arch. Neurol. Psychiat.*, *59*, 559

Weddell, G., Sinclair, D. C. and Feindel, W. H. (1948). An anatomical basis for alterations in quality of pain sensibility. *J. Neurophysiol.*, *11*, 99

White, J. C., Garrey, W. E. and Atkins, J. A. (1933). Cardiac innervation: Experimental and clinical studies. *A.M.A. Arch. Surg.*, *26*, 765

White, J. C. and Selverstone, B. (1956). Pain and related phenomena, including causalgia. Ch. VI in: Woodhall, B. and Beebe, G. W. (eds.) *Peripheral Nerve Regeneration: a Follow-up Study of 3,656 World War II Injuries*. Veterans Administration Medical Monograph, Washington, D.C., Government Printing Office, pp. 311–347

White, J. C., Smithwick, R. H. and Simeone, F. A. (1952). *The Autonomic Nervous System: Anatomy, Physiology and Surgical Application*. 3rd ed., New York, The Macmillan Co., 569 pp.

White, J. C. and Sweet, W. H. (1969). *Pain and the Neurosurgeon: A Forty-Year Experience*. Springfield, Illinois: Charles C. Thomas, 1000 pp.

Youmans, J. R., editor (1973). *Neurological Surgery*. Philadelphia, London, Toronto: W. B. Saunders. Section XII, Pain, in Vol. 3, pp. 1587–1789

6

Chemical Neurolysis in the Treatment of Chronic Pain

Stanley A. Feldman

Divinum est opus sedare dolorum

(*Hippocrates*)

Pain is a subjective concept — to feel pain therefore necessitates an appreciation of what constitutes pleasant and unpleasant sensations. The concept of pain as an unpleasant sensation would appear to be part of the behavioral pattern of many animals, and thus an untrained animal will try to escape from the pain of an electric shock, excessive heat or cold. Nevertheless, a large proportion of our response to pain is acquired or conditioned by experience or emotion. Thus pain has often been associated with punishment for misdemeanors and is therefore unpleasant.

Measurement of pain
Pain, being a subjective concept, cannot exist in an unconscious or semi-conscious person, although the somatic and visceral responses may still persist. Drugs and other forms of therapy may be effective in alleviating pain by altering the patient's attitude to the cause of pain, by affecting the background activity of the brain upon which the 'painful' stimuli fall, by reducing the patient's level of consciousness by providing distraction or by actually lessening the frequency of discharge of the receptors to the pain, or by a combination of any of these. As a result it is often impossible to be certain about the way in which any specific therapeutic effort has produced its effect; it is this very difficulty that makes the objective assessment of any treatment difficult and generalization impossible.

For example, the success of percussion therapy in the treatment of amputation stump pain may be a result of a

157

physical alteration in the tissues surrounding the cut end of the nerve, or, by causing adaptation of the nerve endings and so lessening the frequency of discharge, or, by stimulating large fibers it may close the 'gate' to the pain impulses. Alternatively, its success may be due to the distraction this form of therapy provides to the patient.

Beecher (1946) pointed out how difficult was the objective assessment of pain in battle casualties. Frequently wounds obtained in the heat of battle would only hurt once the battle ended or the injury necessitated removal of the victim from the field of battle. This observation has been confirmed by others. S. Sykes (1961) records examples of injuries occurring in moments of stress which have not produced sensations of pain. He tells of David Livingstone being mauled by a lion in 1872. Whilst the lion mauled at his arm, breaking his humerus, he felt no fear or pain. His only feeling was one of intense curiosity as to which part of his body the lion would undertake next! Another report of Sir E. R. Colborne Bradford (1836–1911) records that when he was seized and mauled by a tiger he felt no pain whilst it was munching his arm. Thus, whilst the response of infants and animals leads us to believe that pain is part of innate behavior pattern and our response to it is instinctive, there is no doubt that conditioning and suggestion can influence our interpretation of this sensation. To the person who expects pain or punishment the sensation will be exaggerated and the somatic response will be great. To the zealot and the person in whom this association is minimized because of pressing environmental distractions, physical discomfort may not produce an emotional response associated with pain.

PAIN THRESHOLD
Bonica (1953) defines the pain threshold as being the lowest perceptible intensity of pain, caused by a powerful stimulus, necessary to induce a sensation of pain. Various methods exist to detect the pain threshold to a variety of different stimuli such as heat, pressure, hyperemia, electric shock, etc. There seems little doubt from studies with these instruments that the pain threshold varies from individual to individual and in the same individual at different times, as a result of exertion, fatigue and distraction. In general, women have a lower pain threshold

than men (Sherman, 1943; Wilder, 1940). Latin and Jewish patients are believed to have a lower pain threshold than African, Indian and N. European peoples. Sherman, 1943, found that 75% of coal miners studied were hyposensitive compared with controls. Other factors that have been shown to influence the pain threshold include mental and physical fatigue and emotional disturbances. Thus the patient who has anxieties about domestic problems, and those who have disturbed sleepless nights, frequently have a reduced tolerance to pain. Because of the variety of factors that may affect the patient's pain threshold it is not surprising that a patient suffering from chronic pain will find the intensity of the pain fluctuating. This does not necessarily reflect alteration in the pathological process producing the sensation but an alteration in the interpretive modality.

GENERAL PRINCIPLES OF TREATMENT

Pain has been considered as a physiological symptom and as such is a manifestation of underlying disease. The contribution of the pathological process, the cerebral interpretation of this process and the environmental contribution will vary from patient to patient and from time to time. It therefore follows that any attempt to treat the presenting symptom of pain without an assessment of the cause is as dangerous as labelling the patient's pain as 'psychological' without first determining that organic pathology of a remediable nature does not exist.

The first principle of the treatment of pain by drugs and by chemical neurolysis is accurate diagnosis and patient assessment. It cannot be emphasized too strongly that symptomatic treatment of pain should not be attempted without having first made a diagnosis of the cause of the symptom. Under these circumstances, the usefulness of local anesthetic nerve blocks as a diagnostic tool is fully justified. It is imperative however that the patient should be told that the effect of the injection of the local anesthetic will be short lived and that it will be more complete than the expected action of the neurolytic agent. Failure to inform the patient may result in an irreparable loss of confidence in the treatment. Should a local anesthetic solution be used to test the suitability for a pain block, complete recovery of sensation should be achieved before the definitive block is attempted.

In this chapter it is intended to deal with pain arising from pathological processes for which there is no specific remedy either due to the nature of the disease process or the inability of the patient to tolerate the treatment. For example, the pain of advanced malignant disease involving the nerve roots in the spinal canal, or of acute pancreatitis, cannot be effectively treated by surgery but can be ameliorated by chemical neurolysis. The pain of intermittent claudication can usually be relieved by surgical intervention to overcome the blockage of the femoral artery. Unfortunately many patients presenting with this symptom have generalized degenerative arterial disease which renders them unfit for major surgery: such patients can be offered symptomatic relief by means of lumbar paravertebral nerve blocks.

The symptomatic treatment of pain necessitates treatment of the patient as a complete person in relationship to his environment. This is best achieved in a pain clinic environment where the physician or surgeon attending the patients can participate in the planning of his overall treatment. The reinforcing effect of mental stress upon the subjective appreciation of pain necessitates consideration of patient anxieties and emotional tensions insofar as these are possible. This cannot be achieved unless the physician treating the pain is prepared to listen to the patient's history carefully and sympathetically and to establish rapport with the patient. It is essential that psychological support should be available for these patients and wherever indicated anti-depressant drugs and tranquilizers should be administered in fully effective doses. Where a patient has been receiving anti-depressant drugs or analgesics prior to treatment it is unwise to discontinue this treatment or even to indicate to the patient that a successful outcome of the treatment is likely to diminish his need for these drugs. It has been the author's experience that unless the patient has experienced dysphoric symptoms from drug therapy it is unwise to anticipate sudden reduction in the need for analgesic drugs. Indeed if drugs with a positive euphoric action are suddenly denied to the patient it is unlikely that his pain will be completely relieved by any other treatment he receives.

Chemical neurolysis and other anesthetic techniques involve inducing a permanent change in the modality of sensory input to the brain, and they may also cause some degree of permanent motor and autonomic disturbance. Because of these major disadvantages it should never be undertaken for trivial or tolerable pain, or for pain that can be easily controlled by moderate doses of non-addictive analgesics. It is strongly indicated in those patients in whom pain can only be controlled by a narcotic dosage that impairs their awareness and depresses their respiration and cough reflex, especially if the pathological condition renders recovery impossible. Many of these patients can be returned to a useful, if limited, life by reducing their pain and improving the quality of their life. Between these two types of patients there remain those in whom severe pain reduces the quality of their life to an unacceptable extent. It is in these patients that generalizations are impossible and in whom the advantage of pain relief must be weighed carefully against the complications that might be induced. Each patient must be regarded separately for assessment of his suitability for a nerve block. In helping to assess these patients it is useful to consider:

(a) Their expectation of life; thus one would be more willing to accept a minor degree of motor weakness or sexual impotence as the price for the relief of pain in a patient in whom the disease process was of itself going to limit his useful ambulant life.

(b) The nature of the patient's occupation and hobbies. Anesthesia, muscle weakness or frequency of micturition may more seriously handicap some patients than others and so adversely affect the quality of their life.

(c) The temporal nature of the pain. It is often useful to have the patient assess the severity of his own pain in each of the four 6-hourly periods of the day using a simple 1–10 scale. Pain which does not prevent his normal physical activities is scaled 1–5, that which renders him bed- or chair-bound, 5–10. By this means it is not uncommon to find that a patient who complains of 'desperate pain' is not being physically limited by it, except for a few hours a day— usually in the evening. In such patients it would be unwise to embark on any method of pain relief that might in itself cause an even greater limitation of his physical activities.

There are certain generalizations to be made about pain relief and especially chemical neurolysis.

1. It must be appreciated that pain is a symptom and that relief of pain itself leaves the underlying condition untreated. It is always preferable *to treat the cause of the pain rather than the symptoms*.

2. Analgesic and specific remedies, such as carbamazepine (Tegretol) in the treatment of trigeminal neuralgia, are preferable to chemical neurolysis as their actions are completely and rapidly reversible whilst the effects of neurolysis may take many months or even years to recover. It is only when the drugs themselves interfere with the quality of the patient's life that other treatment should be tried. When simple analgesics such as dihydro-codeine or paracetamol fail to give relief and opiates have to be used to control the pain — with the consequent hazards of drowsiness, clouding of consciousness, respiratory depression and addiction — chemical neurolysis or surgical treatment of the pain should be considered.

3. If chemical neurolysis is indicated, it should be attempted initially as far peripherally as possible. It is preferable to perform a nerve block at the periphery rather than to block the nerve in the epidural or paravertebral space. It is generally safer to perform a paravertebral block than an epidural block. Similarly, the risks of complications are less with epidural neurolysis than with the administration of drugs intrathecally. Unfortunately, the more central block is often more successful than a peripheral one in the treatment of chronic pain and ultimately one is often forced to use intrathecal injections for prolonged control of chronic pain.

4. Nerve blocks — especially those around the spinal canal — should never be performed in patients receiving anticoagulant therapy.

Agents available for chemical neurolysis

ETHYL ALCOHOL

Ethyl alcohol was the original and is possibly still the most widely used agent for permanent chemical neurolysis. Following intrathecal injection alcohol will cause destruction of both the axons and the myelin sheaths of nerves (Katz, 1970). However, Bonica (1953) suggested that sensory fibers are preferentially destroyed if concentrations of alcohol below 50% are used. Absolute alcohol is hypobaric with a specific gravity of 0.807 compared to 1.007 for CSF and as a result it floats if given intrathecally. It is this hypobaric property that allows the spread of intrathecal alcohol to be limited to the desired spinal segments by careful posturing of the patients. Alcohol neuritis occurs in about 10% of patients who receive this drug for peripheral nerve block, but the incidence appears to be lower when it is injected into the subarachnoid space than when nerve trunk or paravertebral block is attempted. The duration of effect of the neurolysis produced by alcohol varies from a few days to one year or more.

PHENOL

The use of aqueous phenol or phenol in Myodil (iodophendylate) for nerve blocks in strengths of 5–10% gives good analgesia. Owing to its more rapid spread in the aqueous phase there is less necessity for accurate localization of the nerve than with alcohol. For example, if a lumbar sympathetic block is attempted using alcohol injections in the paravertebral space at least three injections at L_1, L_2 and L_3 are required. If aqueous phenol or phenol in myodil is used, one injection will suffice as the drugs flow freely if it is in the correct tissue plane (Figure 6.1). Peripheral nerve blocks with aqueous phenol are not as profound as when alcohol is used and their effect is generally shortlived, anesthesia disappearing in 12 hours and pain often returning in under 1 week. However, in a minority of patients the relief is more permanent.

The use of phenol in glycerine results in a limit to the spread of the phenol as the drug is slowly given up from the glycerine to the aqueous phase. As a result the neurolysis is more complete and localized. Used intrathecally, in 5% concentration, it will give as consistent pain relief as alcohol (Mark et al., 1962). Like alcohol, the neurolytic effect of phenol appears to be indiscriminate and not restricted to sensory nerves (Nathan, 1965).

Phenol in glycerine and phenol in myodil are viscid fluids

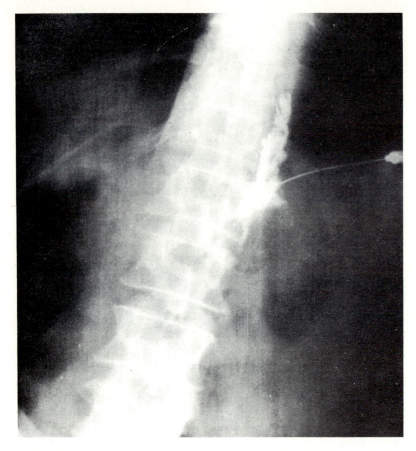

Figure 6.1   Illustrating the spread of phenol in myodil in the paravertebral space

and are strongly hyperbaric S.G. 1.25. They fall to the most dependent site when introduced into the CSF. It is difficult to inject phenol in glycerine solution through a 21 gauge spinal needle unless it is rendered less viscid by warming the ampule in hot water.

Other solutions used to produce neurolysis include 20% ammonium sulphate (Dam, 1965), saline and hypertonic saline, and chlorocresol in glycerine. However none of these chemicals appears to offer substantial advantages over phenol and alcohol, although a recent comparison of chlorocresol in glycerine and phenol in glycerine gave encouraging results (Swerdlow, 1973).

Phenol, alcohol and chlorocresol are far from perfect drugs as they are non-specific in their actions. A drug that was specific for nerve tissue would be preferable if it had little systemic toxicity. In general, it is unfortunate that the drugs that are most effective in producing good pain relief are also those that cause the highest incidence of neurological side effects.

SIDE EFFECTS

All the solutions used for chemical neurolysis are non-specific protein poisons and as such are likely to affect all tissues with which they come in contact causing cell death and reactionary fibrosis. This late fibrosis may cause secondary symptoms if complete sensory destruction has not been achieved. This is particularly likely to occur when alcohol is used but has also been reported following application of phenol.

The main complication of chemical neurolysis is anesthesia, hyperesthesia and motor weakness. Even in the most experienced hands a 10% incidence of significant side effects of this nature have been recorded (Kuzucu *et al.*, 1966). In the author's experience the incidence of minor undesirable side effects — such as transient skin anesthesia, hyperalgesia around the area blocked and overt, even though temporary, muscle or sphincter paralysis — has been 15–20% following 5% intrathecal phenol in glycerine injection. Permanent muscle weakness or sphincter difficulty is acceptably low, being most obvious in those patients, usually with terminal cancer, in whom the risk has been considered to be acceptable. Nevertheless the distress caused by these sequelae are sufficient to mitigate against the use of this technique, except when all other treatments have failed. Probably the most unsatisfactory aspect of this form of therapy is the unpredictable nature of the patient's response. Thus one patient may develop permanent muscle weakness and anesthesia with a dose of subarachnoid phenol that produced no demonstrable effect in another patient. In general a patient who is resistant to phenol on one occasion will remain resistant at all times and if subsequent blocks are required it is preferable to use alcohol.

Pain associated with somatic peripheral nerves

(a) *Due to irritation or disease of somatic nerves*
This is a common presentation of pain which may be due to a
variety of different causes such as sciatica which may be due to
intervertebral disc lesions, nerve entrapment in scar tissue, pain
due to stretching of nerves or pressure on nerves, to herpes
zoster, amputation stump neuromas and due to carcinatomous
involvement of the nerve, trunk or its root by deposits in the
vertebrae.

(b) *Due to disease of tissues supplied by somatic nerves*
In addition to these pains are those due to tissue trauma in the
areas supplied by a particular somatic nerve. Pain due to
trauma or carcinoma involving the neck, chest wall, pleura,
etc., will be carried along the appropriate somatic nerve serving
that dermatome.

(c) *Pain referred to a somatic dermatome*
Pain due to inflammation, tumor or ischemia involving the
viscera may be referred to a somatic dermatome. Thus sub-
diaphragmatic inflammation may present as shoulder tip pain
and arm pain may be due to myocardial ischemia. Girdle
pains may be due to the late effects of Herpes zoster. All these
pains have certain features in common:

1. Their distribution is limited to an anatomical dermatome pattern (see Figure 6.2).

2. Interruption of the nerve by local analgesics or by
neurolysis will alleviate the symptoms. Obviously this will be
more effective if the causal agent is distal to the point of nervous
interruption, but it will usually give some relief even in cases
where the nerve is subject to irritation in the spinal cord and
the block is performed on the peripheral nerve. Thus the pain
of acute sciatica may often be partially alleviated by a sciatic
nerve block. However, the results are seldom complete and very
short lived. Similarly infiltration of local anesthetic solution
will usually alleviate referred pain. For example the pain of
severe dysmenorrhea can frequently be relieved by infiltration with 1% lignocaine subcutaneously over the symphysis
pubis.

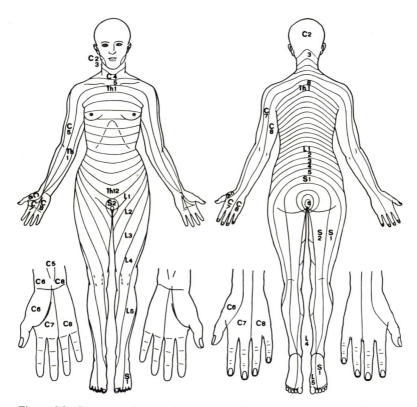

Figure 6.2 Dermatome innervation of the skin. Pain of an organic nature will usually be distributed in an anatomical dermatome pattern

TREATMENT

All these pains are amenable to some form of neurolysis. Widespread pain (more than 3 dermatomes), or a bilateral involvement lessens the chances of complete relief of pain without permanent numbness or weakness. In such cases it is wise to perform the block in two or more sessions at monthly intervals.

If a peripheral nerve block is performed with either aqueous phenol or alcohol, accurate localization of the nerve is essential. If paresthesia cannot be elicited on insertion of the needle, electrical stimulation of the needle may help to localize the nerve and by reproducing the pain, indicate the

most advantageous site for injection. This can easily be performed using a simple peripheral nerve stimulator. If the nature
of the disease makes peripheral nerve block impossible, epidural or subarachnoid block may be required. The exact site of
spinal puncture will depend upon the vertebral level at which
the appropriate nerve root is given off from the spinal cord.
This is 1–2 vertebral segments higher than the spinal level in
the cervical and thoracic regions, and 2–3 vertebral segments
higher in the lumbar region, whilst sacral blocks are achieved
by a spinal tap at L_2–L_3, allowing the solution to flow down
around the cauda equina, by having the patient sitting upright
if a hyperbaric is used, and in the knee elbow position if alcohol
is used. In general, it is preferable to use the minimum volume
of the weakest solution to be effective in the first instance, and
to repeat the block if the pain recurs. Unfortunately, it is often
difficult to perform repeated blocks at frequent intervals due
to the difficulty in obtaining a ready flow of CSF. If phenol in
glycerine or absolute alcohol is used the spinal needle may be
left *in situ* whilst 0.1 ml increments are given until there is
complete pain relief. In this way, the neurolysis may be
titrated against the pain. In order that this can be achieved the
previous 6 hours' dosages of analgesics should be omitted. It is
surprising how frequently, even if no analgesics have been
administered, the patient's pain will be minimal when he
presents for nerve block. Presumably the attention and anticipation reduces the symptoms.

COMPLICATIONS
1. *Incomplete pain relief.* This is common and is an indication for
a repeat of the block with a slightly larger volume of solution
or a stronger concentration of phenol. The volume of phenol
should not be increased by more than 50% nor should the total
amount administered intrathecally exceed 1.5 ml at one sitting.
    2. *Neuralgia.* This occurs in about 10% of all alcohol peri-
pheral nerve blocks. If it is mild it should be treated with sedatives. If severe, the block should be repeated to achieve complete
neurolysis.
    3. *Anesthesia.* This is likely to diminish with time. It is often
an unavoidable side effect, and the price paid for a complete
pain relief. The anesthetic area is frequently surrounded by a

zone of hypesthesia which may be very uncomfortable. Facial anesthesia is especially troublesome.

4. *Bladder sphincter incontinence and constipation.* These complications of lower lumbar and sacral blocks are very troublesome. Some recovery can usually be expected. To avoid these complications, patients suffering from lubo-sacral pains should be postured to ensure only unilateral neurolysis and the block should not be repeated on the other side in under 3 weeks. It can generally be avoided if less than 0.5 ml of alcohol or 0.7 ml of 5% phenol in glycerine is used together with careful posture to ensure neurolysis limited to a restricted region of the most dependent part of the thecal sac. Alternatively, it may be avoided by performing trans sacral nerve blocks (paravertebral) by injecting the solution through the posterior sacral foramena. Unfortunately, this treatment is less effective against the sacral and coccygeal pain of pelvic carcinoma.

Treatment of specific conditions

Illustrative of the approach to the use of chemical neurolysis.

1. NERVE IRRITATION

(a) *Nerve entrapment*

This condition is most frequently observed following repair of an inguinal hernia when the ilio-hypogastric nerve becomes trapped in scar tissue associated with the repair. It demonstrates the features of pain associated with a limited distribution. The pain is constant in position, radiates from the trapped area distally, can be partially relieved by the injection of local anesthetic over the area of its distribution and completely relieved by the injection of local anesthetic proximal to, or at the site of, the irritation. The condition responds well to the injection of 2 ml of 7.5% aqueous phenol at the site of the entrapment. The exact injection site can be localized using electrical faradic stimulation through the injection needle. When the nerve has been positively identified by these means stimulation will reproduce the pain. Phenol should not be injected immediately after a local anesthetic solution as the volume of the local anesthetic will cause dilution. If a local anesthetic solution has been used as a diagnostic test, 6 hours should elapse and sensation restored before the definitive phenol block is performed.

(b) *Rib injuries*

Injuries involving the chest wall are exceedingly common especially as a result of deceleration car accidents. The pain may be due to severe bruising and contusion of the chest wall, or if severe and localized, due to rib fracture. These pains can be adequately treated by analgesics and by application of a suitable elastic bandage that limits movement. Unfortunately in some patients with multiple rib injuries, the restriction of movement that results from the pain and the strapping, combined with respiratory depression and diminished activity of the cough reflex that result from the use of analgesics produces pulmonary atelectasis. This is especially likely to occur in older patients and in heavy smokers. In these patients repeated subcostal blocks or the introduction of a catheter into the epidural space and the use of segmental analgesia allows them to breathe deeply without pain and to cough up sputum.

In general it is preferable to perform subcostal nerve blocks three times a day for the two or three days following the accident than to use segmental epidural anesthesia with its possible complications. However, if more than three ribs require blocking, an epidural anesthetic should be considered.

Subcostal nerve block

This is an extremely easy and safe nerve block to perform if the area to be blocked is anterior to the posterior axillary line. The subcostal nerve runs in the subcostal groove adjacent to the artery. The rib associated with the nerve to be blocked is identified and a needle inserted under its lower border. A syringe should be attached to the needle lest the pleural cavity be inadvertently entered and a pneumothorax induced by air entering through the open end of the needle. As the needle slips below the rib, 3 ml of 2% lignocaine or 0.5% bupivacaine is injected after ascertaining by aspiration that the tip of the needle is not in a blood vessel. By this means satisfactory analgesia can be obtained for about 3–6 hours.

More perfect analgesia is afforded by a segmental epidural block. This is achieved by inserting a catheter into the epidural space and advancing its tip to a level 1 dermatome above the area of the pain. 8 ml of 0.5% bupivacaine injected through the catheter will produce pain relief over 3 to 4 dermatomes for 4–6 hours. If wider areas are to be blocked, larger volumes of bupivacaine or lignocaine will be required and there is a greater risk of hypotension from the widespread sympathetic paralysis that results. It is advisable therefore to have the patient semirecumbent when the injection is made and to have ready access to a vein. Should hypotension occur, the patient should be placed flat and 500–1,000 ml of electrolyte solution should be infused.

2. FACIAL PAINS (EXCLUDING MIGRAINE)
Migraine pain is not amenable to chemical neurolysis and should be treated by specific therapy.

Facial neuralgias
Of these the most frequent and most incapacitating is trigeminal neuralgia. The etiology of this condition is unknown and specific therapy is not available. Fortunately many patients, except those with long standing pain, respond well to a drug regime of carbamazepine (Tegretol) either alone or in combination with sodium phenytoin 0.1 g twice daily. Carbamazepine 200 mg should be administered starting with one tablet a day, increasing up to eight a day if the pain is unrelieved at a lesser dose level. Those patients who are refractory to this treatment and in whom the pain is severe should be considered for either chemical neurolysis or surgery.

The dangers involved in trigeminal neurectomy are those of paralysis of the motor roots to the jaw muscles and of the loss of corneal sensation with consequent risk of corneal ulceration. These risks are lessened at surgery by removing only the lower two-thirds of the nerve roots and by identifying the motor branch so that it can be preserved. Temporary chemical interruption of one or more branches of the trigeminal nerve by local anesthetic solutions or by Gasserian ganglion block is an effective technique for use in the differential diagnosis of refractory facial pains. By using phenol or alcohol, long termed neurolysis is produced for the treatment of trigeminal neuralgia.

It is simpler and safer than surgical neurectomy but probably less reliable.

As with all nerve blocks it is preferable to attempt to interrupt the nerve as peripherally as possible. Thus for pain affecting the maxillary and mandibular divisions of the V nerve it is preferable to perform a separate maxillary and mandibular block than to proceed to Gasserian block as a primary treatment. Mandibular V block is simple to perform by inserting a needle at right angles to skin through the zygomatic notch into the pterygoid fossa where the nerve emerges from the foramen ovale. A test injection of local anesthesia (1% ligocaine) will produce anesthesia of the lower jaw, lingual and inferior dental nerve distribution (see Figure 6.3). If a permanent effect is required, 3 ml 6–8% aqueous phenol should be injected. This very satisfactory block is extremely useful for controlling pain limited to the 3rd division of the trigeminal nerve, but its effects are seldom prolonged beyond 1–2 years. The main complication of this block is that of a hematoma, which besides being temporarily painful and unsightly, will also mitigate against the success of the block. Although useful for some cases of trigeminal neuralgia, it is especially indicated for painful tumors of mandibular alveolus and lower lip, and it will often successfully relieve the distressing trismus associated with these conditions.

Maxillary V

Various approaches have been described to reach this nerve as it lies in the pterygo-palatine fossa after emerging from the foramen rotundum. The anterior approach in front of the ramus of the mandible is probably the simplest and least disturbing to the conscious patient. A successful block of this nerve results in cessation of any painful sensation emanating from the maxillary antrum, upper teeth, tonsils, lip and gums, or the lower part of the nose. This block is useful in the differential diagnosis of atypical facial pains. It is of therapeutic value in the treatment of some forms of trigeminal neuralgia and it is especially useful in relieving the pain of malignant infiltrating cancer of the antrum. As with mandibular V block its effects are less long-lasting than Gasserian ganglion block.

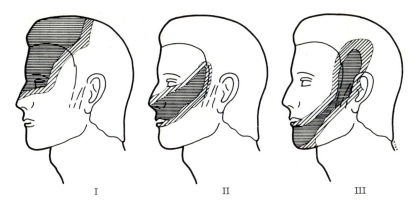

Figure 6.3   The limits of anesthesia achieved by blocking (I) (Ophthalmic) V nerve division, (II) (Maxillary) V nerve division, (III) (Mandibular) V nerve division

Ophthalmic V

Orbital nerve block is seldom indicated for the relief of pain although used frequently to facilitate ophthalmic surgery. Although the ethmoidal branch of the ophthalmic nerve is commonly involved in malignant tumors of the maxilla it is unsafe to block this nerve with neurolytic agents owing to its proximity to the ophthalmic nerve and the fear of causing visual disturbance or blindness. The supraorbital nerve is commonly involved in trigeminal neuralgia, and indeed supraorbital pain may be the only, or the most persistent symptom of this condition. In these patients block of the supraorbital nerve with 1% lignocaine as it runs over the orbital ridge is useful in the diagnosis and in planning treatment. Alcohol or aqueous phenol block of the supraorbital nerve will cause prolonged relief of neuralgia in most patients although the effect is seldom permanent and may have to be repeated.

The majority of cases of trigeminal neuralgia can be adequately treated either by drugs or by a combination of drug therapy and nerve block of a branch of the V nerve involved in the disease. Only if this fails is Gasserian ganglion block justified.

Gasserian ganglion block

This block is best performed under x-ray control using an image intensifier. The needle is introduced below the posterior

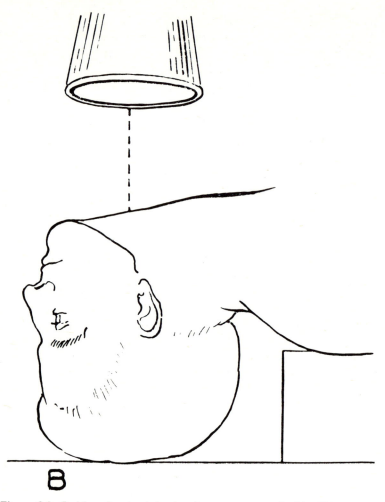

Figure 6.4 Position of patient's head and x-ray apparatus for identifying a needle entering the foramen ovale for Gasserian ganglion block

third of the zygoma opposite the 2nd upper molar tooth. The needle is passed postero-medially and in an upward direction. The needle passes behind the pterygoid plate to the foramen ovale. At this point it is useful to identify the foramen using x-ray control. The best position for this is with the neck fully extended and a sandbag under the patient's shoulders (Figure 6.4). As the needle is introduced through the foramen, mandibular paresthesiae are usual. The needle is advanced 1 cm into the cave of Meckel, in which lies the ganglion. Aspiration through the needle is essential to establish that it is still extradural, and this should be confirmed by the injection of 1 ml of myodil. If the needle is in the correct position 0.5 to 0.75 ml of alcohol or 1 ml of phenol in myodil (5%) should be injected. If the needle is intrathecal, injection of phenol or alcohol should not be attempted.

Inadvertent leakage of agents into the CSF may cause facial or ocular paralysis and is especially to be avoided. Hyperalgesia and numbness are occasionally troublesome immediate sequelae but they are seldom long lasting.

The technique of Gasserian ganglion block with alcohol or phenol is a very satisfactory treatment for trigeminal neuralgia in most people. Although according to Moore (1957) the failure rate is in the order of 25%, the use of the image intensifier since his report has reduced this failure rate in most centers to 10%. The incidence of corneal anesthesia is reported to be higher after the use of alcohol (Moore, 1957) who emphasizes the advantages of treating the divisions of the V nerve rather than performing a Gasserian ganglion block.

Occipital neuralgia (cervico-capital neuralgia)
This is a painful and common condition. It presents as a lancinating pain passing from the nape of the neck toward the vertex of the skull. The condition is usually unilateral and the pain may spread to other areas of the head or to the ear.

There are many potential causes of the pain. The commonest is due to a fibrositic reaction of the tendinous portion of the trapezius muscle which involves the occipital nerve as it penetrates the muscle. Fibrositic nodules can often be palpated and the injection of a short acting local anesthetic into these nodules may produce long lasting relief. It is recommended that hydrocortisone should be included with the local anesthetic to obtain the best results. It is important to ensure that the neuralgia is not the result of traumatic displacement of the vertebra or by cervical osteoarthritis.

3. BACK PAINS

Lumbar epidural block
The treatment of acute back pain with associated muscle spasm by means of an epidural injection of dilute local anesthetic solution often has a dramatic effect in terminating these incapacitating pains. Whilst the mechanism underlying the success of this treatment is uncertain, it would seem reasonable to assume that its basis lies in the relief of the pain by the epidural anesthetic and the relaxation of the intense muscle spasm which disturbs the spinal posture maintaining the painful state.

Owing to the intense discomfort of this condition the patient should be sedated or anesthetized for the actual epidural injection. Most operators use 20–30 ml of 0.5% lignocaine with or without methylprednisolone or hydrocortisone to achieve amelioration of the pain without overt motor weakness. The injection is usually given at the L_{2-3} or L_{3-4} interspace. Following the injection the patient is encouraged to move freely and to perform moderate back exercises. Burn in 1973 reported a high success rate with epidural block together with back manipulation under general anesthesia. In the author's experience, immediate and permanent relief of pain is achieved in over 50% of patients following the first injection and a further 20–25% of patients are improved following a second injection. The longer the pain has been present before the patient comes for treatment, the lower the success rate. The most dramatic successes with this technique are in those patients who have a sudden acute back strain within the previous 48 hours.

The treatment of chronic back pains associated with limited straight leg raising and evidence of intervertebral disc disease, including patients in whom laminectomy has failed to relieve their symptoms, is less rewarding but nevertheless worthwhile. A solution of 30 ml of 0.5% lignocaine (or saline) containing methyl prednisolone 50 mg is recommended. Larger volumes of saline with higher doses of steroid have been proposed but they do not appear to produce significantly better results and may be dangerous due to the transient increase in CSF pressure produced. Although less than 50% of patients receive more than temporary relief from this treatment it is worth repeating two or three times in the hope of affecting intravertebral adhesions around nerve roots. As the treatment itself carries little risk and discomfort it is justified in spite of the lower permanent cure rate. The injection of a very large volume of saline, either by the lumbar or caudal epidural route, does not increase the success rate of this form of treatment and may be hazardous.

4. INTERMITTENT CLAUDICATION

This distressingly painful condition predominantly affects elderly males who have been heavy cigarette smokers. In 80% of patients it is associated with a blockage of the femoral artery. Whenever possible arterial reconstructive surgery should be performed as this offers the only real hope of achieving the increased muscle blood flow required by the muscles during exercise. Lumbar sympathectomy may make the symptoms worse by increasing the proportion of blood entering the limb, that is diverted to the skin. If surgical operation to improve the total blood flow to the limb is impracticable because of concomitant disease, debility or failure of adequate 'run off' of blood, then conservative measures to alleviate pain are indicated. The most successful procedure for these patients is lumbar paravertebral block of their somatic nerves at a level of L_{1-2-3}. This is performed using an x-ray image intensifier to demonstrate the tip of the needle on the lateral surface of the lumbar vertebra. A single injection of 5–7 ml of 7.5% phenol in myodil or 10% aqueous phenol at L_2 which spreads in the psoas sheath affecting the lumbar plexus (Figure 6.5) is sufficient to cause prolonged relief of claudicant pain. In the author's series of some 65 patients treated in this manner, 90% of patients receiving the nerve block more than doubled their claudication distance within 12 hours. At the end of 12 to 18 months some 45% of patients had maintained some degree of improvement.

5. TREATMENT OF VASOSPASTIC STATES

Painful vasospasm of the vessels of the limbs may follow trauma to limb or embolism in the artery of that limb. However, in a number of patients it appears to be idiopathic. These

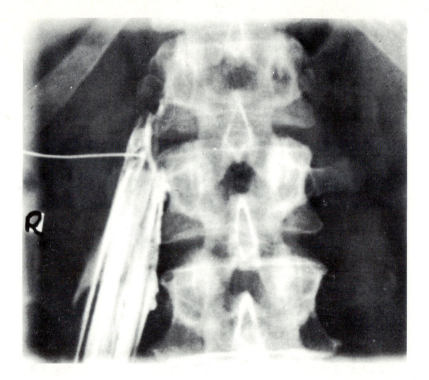

Figure 6.5 Lumbar somatic nerve block for treatment of intermittent claudication. The phenol in myodil spreads out into the psoas sheath affecting the lumbar plexus

symptoms respond dramatically to autonomic nerve block of the sympathetic outflow to the limb concerned.

Lumbar sympathetic block
This is best achieved by means of a paravertebral injection with the point of the needle resting on the antero lateral surface of L_2 vertebral body. Seven to 10 ml of 7.5% phenol in myodil or 10% aqueous phenol is injected (Figure 6.1). The myodil demonstrates the typical spread of the phenol up and down the vertebral bodies, which occurs if the injection is in the correct tissue plane. The sign of a successful block is an improvement in skin temperature (this may take 24 hours to reach its maximum) and a relief of painful symptoms.

Stellate ganglion block

This simple block is extremely useful in relieving acute pain of vasospastic states in the hand and *causalgic pains* in wrist and arm. Because of the tendency of any neurolytic solution to trickle down the pleura and cause pain, it is preferable to use local ancsthetic solutions only. If a permanent result is desired the judicious use of alcohol may be attempted after previously warning the patient of possible pleural pain, but the author prefers to advise surgical sympathectomy for these patients. Complications of this block include pneumothorax (bilateral blocks should never be attempted at one sitting), phrenic nerve paresis and inadvertent intrathecal injection. The block is performed using an intramuscular needle (19 SWG) which is inserted medial to the sternal head of sternomastoid muscle until it impinges upon the transverse process of the 7th cervical vertebra. This can be palpated in most patients and lies about two fingers' breadths above the sterno-clavicular joint.

Splanchnic nerve block

In many patients with intra-abdominal disease, pain is referred to a somatic dermatomal distribution and block of that dermatome with either a local anesthetic or with phenol or alcohol will produce pain relief. However, under some circumstances the pain relief can only be achieved by widespread nerve block carrying with it the risks of unpleasant side effects. In these patients splanchnic nerve block may be a useful procedure although the quality of pain relief it produces is seldom as complete as with somatic nerve block. Thus the pain of a patient with infiltrating carcinoma of the pancreas may be completely relieved by nerve block of T_{12}–L_1–L_2 and partially relieved by a splanchnic nerve block. Splanchnic nerve block with a local anesthetic is effective in the treatment of the pain of *acute pancreatitis* but again a better quality of pain relief follows the careful positioning of an epidural catheter at T_{12}–L_1 level and the use of a segmental epidural block using 4–8 ml of 0.25% bupivacaine 4–6 hourly.

The less circumscribed abdominal pain associated with *porphyria* is said to respond well to a splanchnic nerve block.

Splanchnic nerve block is best performed with the patient prone. A 9 in, 21 SWG needle is used and introduced from a point 5–8 cm from the midline with the point directed onto the anterolateral aspect of the 1st lumbar vertebra. Once this bony landmark is reached a depth mark should be set and the needle advanced a further 2–3 cm into the fossa around the great vessels. The block is most safely and easily performed with the aid of an image intensifier and x-ray apparatus. Once the needle is in place 1–2 ml of myodil injected through the needle will indicate the likely spread of any anesthetic solution administered.

6. POST-HERPETIC NEURALGIA

This condition is extremely difficult to treat. Because the pain is of a non-malignant nature one is reluctant to resort to the use of spinothalamic tractotomy or intrathecal injection of phenol in glycerine or alcohol yet, in the author's experience in established post herpetic pain, the pain is seldom relieved by less hazardous treatments. Some authors (Moore, 1957) claim success with sympathetic blocks in the treatment of this condition — indicating a causalgic nature of the pain — whilst others have reported some success with repeated local infiltrations if the pain is of short duration (Bonica, 1953). Both these treatments are worthy of trial before resorting to chemical neurolysis. Large doses of vitamin B complex, deep x-ray therapy and intravenous procaine have largely been abandoned. A common complication of the use of intrathecal or epidural injection of phenol in the treatment of these patients is the development of a zone of hyperalgesia around the area blocked. It is essential to use the minimal dose of phenol or alcohol possible in the treatment of this condition. It is preferable to repeat an inadequate block on two or three occasions rather than to leave a large area of numbness and a zone of hyperalgesia in these patients. A recently introduced treatment which has given promising results is to remove the area of affected skin surgically and to undercut the adjacent skin so as to denervate the affected area.

Amputation stump pain and phantom limb pain

Failure to distinguish these two separate conditions results in maltreatment. However, it is possible for both forms of pain to coincide.

STUMP PAIN

Following amputation, stump pain may develop at any time from weeks to months after the operation. The cause of the pain varies from a painful keloid scar, ulceration of the skin owing to a bad fitting socket prothesis or the development of a stump neuroma, to a form of claudicant pain associated with the abnormal muscular exertion necessary to utilize a short stump as a lever to move a long heavy prosthesis. The claudicant type pain can be aggravated by pre-existing vascular disease and by the loss of a variable resistance effect of the skin and muscles of the leg which normally control blood flow through the limb. As a result of the loss of this controlling system the blood 'run off' from an amputation stump is often low and has little ability to vary according to the metabolic needs of the stump.

Painful scars and stump neuromas should be dealt with surgically. If pain recurs after excision of a painful scar or stump neuroma, percussion therapy may be tried. Enthusiastic reports of the success of this form of treatment suggest that the good results are due to a combination of neurological and psychological effects. Bad fitting limb prostheses can similarly be corrected. Other pains, including claudicant type pains, rest pain in stump and bursting sensations can be treated by lumbar paravertebral block of both somatic and sympathetic nerves.

Unfortunately, the results of these ill understood pains are not as good as with other chronic pains and the possibility has to be considered that many patients reject their prostheses for one of many reasons unconnected with true pathology and which manifest as stump pain.

PHANTOM LIMB PAIN

Following amputation of a limb or other major part of the anatomy, phantom phenomena commonly occur. In most patients the condition is short lived and, whilst it is disquieting, it seldom progresses to overt pain. Pain in a phantom limb is not common but is extremely difficult to treat. The pain usually lacks a dermatome or neural distribution and commonly is felt in that part of the limb that was painful at the time of the initial injury. Thus a patient whose foot was crushed prior to amputation tends to feel pain in his toes. The author has had the opportunity to administer spinal and epidural anesthetics to several of these patients and the response of the patient is usually similar. The patient declares that his phantom has 'gone numb and heavy', but in all but one case, the pain remained as intense or even more severe. The single patient whose pain was relieved by the epidural anesthetic had in fact referred pain the $L_1 L_2$ distribution following a painful intramuscular injection into the lateral aspect of the buttock. This patient responded to an L_2 somatic nerve block.

Phantom limb pain is generally not amenable to therapeutic nerve block unless there is a dermatome or neural distribution of the pain.

8. TREATMENT OF TERMINAL CARE PATIENTS

Continuous epidural block
Patients with disseminated disease and widespread pain may often be helped by the use of a continuous epidural block covering the principal segments involved in their pain. By using dilute solutions of bupivacaine (0.25% without adrenaline) it is possible to make many patients sufficiently comfortable to undergo treatments such as radiotherapy without at the same time inducing unpleasant side effects. Although the indications for this form of treatment are limited it can prove to be a most worthwhile practice and has on occasions been continued for up to two months before the patient ultimately died of his disease, having suffered the minimum of discomfort.

TREATMENT OF CHRONIC PAIN BY CSF BARBOTAGE
Barbotage — the alternate withdrawal and replacement of the CSF has been used in the treatment of severe, chronic pain by Lloyd (1972). Originally ice cold saline was used (Hitchcock, 1967) but Lloyd (1972) in his series of 50 patients used the patient's own CSF. In 20 patients the CSF was cooled before being reintroduced intrathecally. 70% of patients had some relief of pain following this procedure, but in some cases it was not prolonged. There appears to be a greater success rate when the barbotage was carried out in the region affected by the pain. Thus thoracic barbotage produced better results for pain

relief in the thoracic region than did the normal lumbar procedure. Cooling the CSF before reintroduction into the theca improved the results when the pain was in the cervical region but not elsewhere. Lloyd suggests that the increased pressure created intrathecally might be the cause of the pain relief, possibly by causing areas of ischemic necrosis. The place of this technique in the treatment of severe chronic pain is probably limited although it appears to warrant further trial, especially for the treatment of pain due to malignant disease, occurring in the lumbar or lumbo-sacral region.

OTHER METHODS OF TREATMENT

Chemical neurolysis is an attractive and useful method of treatment of many forms of chronic pain. However, it is essential that the physician treating pain should remain open to all methods of pain relief and that he should not embrace therapeutic nerve blocks to the exclusion of a consideration of the value of spino-thalamic cordotomy and stimulation of a dorsal root or a large afferent nerve. The recent development of percutaneous cordotomy has rendered spino-thalamic cordotomy quick and relatively safe without the debilitating effect of subjecting the patient to surgery (Lipton, 1968). Unfortunately the long termed results of cordotomy are disappointing and the procedure may have to be repeated at a higher level.

Experience with stimulation of a large afferent nerve or dorsal nerve root (Shealy et al., 1967; Wall and Sweet, 1967) is still too limited to be certain of the ultimate usefulness of this form of therapy which is based upon the 'gate' theory of pain sensation.

The usefulness of prefrontal leucotomy in selected patients should be considered as a final resort in those patients in whom other treatments have failed and in whom a large reactive element is present.

The search for better and more specific treatments for chronic pain has not received the attention it merits and very often the response to therapy by the relatively crude methods available is disappointing. With the better understanding of neurophysiology of pain it is to be hoped that in the future we will be able to base our treatments on a better scientific basis and to understand our failures by an appreciation of the pharmacology of the drugs we use and the neuroanatomy of the pathways we are trying to interrupt.

REFERENCES

Beecher, H. K. (1946). Pain in man wounded in battle. *Ann. Surg.*, *123*, 96

Bonica, J. J. (1953). *The Management of Pain.* London: Henry Kimpton

Burn, J. M. B. (1972). *The treatment of the lumbosciatic syndrome by epidural injection and manipulation under general anaesthesia.* Report to Intractable Pain Soc., Cardiff, England

Dam, W. H. (1965). Therapeutic Blocks. *Acta Chir. Scand.* (Suppl.), *343*, 189

Hitchcock, E. (1967). Hypothermic subarachnoid irrigation for intractable pain. *Lancet*, **i**, 1133

Katz, J. (1970). Pain; *Theory and Management in Scientific Foundations Anaesthesia.* Scurr and Feldman, editors. London: Heinemann

Kuzucu, E. Y., Derrick, W. S. and Wilber, S. A. (1966). Control of intractable pain with subarachnoid alcohol block. *J. Amer. Med. Ass.*, *195*, 541

Lipton, S. (1968). Percutaneous electrical cardotomy in relief of intractable pain. *Brit. Med. J.*, *2*, 210

Lloyd, J. W., Hughes, J. T. and Davies-Jones, G. A. B. (1972). Relief of severe intractable pain by barbotage of cerebrospinal fluid. *Lancet*, **i**, 354

Mark, V. H., White, J. C., Zervas, N. T., Ervin, F. R. and Richardson, E. P. (1962). Intrathecal use of phenol for the relief of chronic pain. *New England J. Med.*, *267*, 589

Moore, D. C. (1957). *Regional Block.* Illinois: Charles C. Thomas

Nathan, P. W., Sears, T. A. and Smith, N. C. (1965). Effects of phenol solution on the nerve roots of the cat. *Neurological Science*, *2*, 7

Shealy, C. N., Taslitz, N., Mortimer, J. T. and Becker, D. P. (1967). Electrical Inhibition of pain; experimental evaluation. *Current Res. Anaesthesia and Analgesia*, *46*, 299

Sherman, E. D. (1943). Sensitivity to pain. *Canadian Med. Ass. J.*, *48*, 437

Swerdlow, M. (1973). Intrathecal chlorocresol: A comparison with phenol in the treatment of intractable pain. *Anaesthesia*, *28*, 297

Sykes, S. (1961). *Essays on the first Hundred Years of Anaesthesia*, Vol. II. London: Livingstone

Wall, P. D. and Sweet, H. W. (1967). Temporary abolition of pain in man. *Science*, *155*, 108

Wilder, R. M. (1940). Sensitivity to pain. *Proc. Mayo Clinic*, *15*, 551

For detailed explanation of methods used in performing therapeutic nerve blocks, see:

1. *Management of Pain* by J. J. Bonica (1953). London: Henry Kimpton Ltd.
2. *Regional Block* by D. C. Moore (1957). Springfield, Illinois: Charles C. Thomas
3. *Intractable Pain* by M. Mehta (1973). W. B. Saunders, London.

Index

185